MOBILISATION TECHNIQUES

John Blackman DO MRO MCSP SRP

Karen Prip DFFMT
Registered Physiotherapist
Chairman of Danish Association of Manual Physiotherapists, Denmark

Foreword by
Gregory P. Grieve FCSP DipTP
Honorary Fellow of the Chartered Society of Physiotherapy;
Founder Member of the Manipulation Association of Chartered Physiotherapists;
Formerly Clinical Tutor, Spinal Treatment Unit, Royal National Orthopaedic Hospital, London,
and Norfolk and Norwich Hospital, Norwich

SECOND EDITION

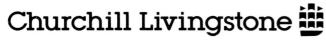

Churchill Livingstone

EDINBURGH LONDON MELBOURNE AND NEW YORK 1988

CHURCHILL LIVINGSTONE
Medical Division of Longman Group UK Limited

Distributed in the United States of America by
Churchill Livingstone Inc., 1560 Broadway,
New York, N.Y. 10036, and by associated
companies, branches and representatives throughout
the world.

First edition 1986
Second edition 1988

ISBN 0-443-03940-2

British Library Cataloguing in Publication Data
Prip, Karen
   Mobilisation techniques. — 2nd ed.
   1. Man. Joints. Manipulation
   I. Title II. Blackman, John
   616.7'20662

Printed in Great Britain by
Butler & Tanner Ltd, Frome and London

FOREWORD

The second edition of this excellent text is a timely and apt expression of the increasing United Kingdom ties with continental Europe. The co-authors, experienced manual therapists and clinical teachers, represent two nations with a Scandinavian rather than a Latin heritage. Both countries are rich in the history of physical treatment for common musculoskeletal conditions. In continuing this tradition the authors have packed much wisdom and good teaching into what they modestly term an 'aide-mémoire' for those with appropriate professional qualifications and suitably specialised training.

Karen Prip is the energetic and much-travelled leader of the Danish Manual Therapy Group, and, as was evident in John Blackman's chapter in *Modern Manual Therapy of the Vertebral Column* (1986), the authors have no particular axe to grind and are interested only in good and effective work. An unusual aspect of this text is that one of the authors stands astride both physiotherapy and osteopathy — a *rara avis* indeed. The confluence of physiotherapy and osteopathy is plain, and this might benefit both professions.

Manual therapy teachers will note some important points, i.e. the photographic illustrations are superb and hand placings are abundantly clear; soft-tissue stretching techniques are included, implying that 'the joint' is not necessarily the prime culprit; there is wise advice about the dangerous fallacy that traction makes manipulations safer.

A selection of both spinal and peripheral joint techniques is featured, including some interesting alternatives for the shoulder, hip, sacro-iliac joints and others.

This unique text cannot fail to appeal to all manual therapists, of whatever persuasion or philosophy.

Halesworth, Suffolk   Gregory P. Grieve

ACKNOWLEDGEMENTS

We would like to express special gratitude to Lene Abildhauge, Aut. Physiotherapist, DFFMT, who was a joint author of the first edition and collaborator for this second edition. In addition she has been a very patient model during long and tedious photographic sessions.

We are also grateful to the following: the Danish Manual Therapy Group who have given great support at all times; Mr Gregory Grieve FCSP, DipTP, for his valued and encouraging advice and for granting us permission to reproduce paragraphs from John Blackman's contribution (Ch. 60) to *Modern Manual Therapy of the Vertebral Column* (Churchill Livingstone, Edinburgh); Bent Balsby, photographer, who has devoted much time, technical skill and enthusiasm to the illustrations; Agnete Karle, Dr med., who has generously provided us with radiographs; and finally Leif Mogensen, consultant in audio-visual aids, for his expertise and help in producing photographic and radiographic prints.

CONTENTS

INTRODUCTION

The recent surge of interest in the subject of joint manipulation has produced the illusion that a bright and glorious new star has appeared in the medical heavens. Nothing could be further from the truth. Treatment by manipulation is as old as mankind; every civilisation and every generation has possessed and cherished its 'bone setters'. Together with the science of herbalism, manipulation provided the foundation for medicine.

It fell to the osteopaths to collect and rationalise the myriad of manipulative techniques into a system of healing. Whether their early physiological arguments were right or wrong, they deserve the credit for guiding the craft of manipulation through the difficult years when it was scorned as quackery. We owe the present state of the art to the courage and determination of the osteopathic profession. Orthodox medicine adopts an ever-recurring attitude to new ideas: first, agressive hostility, followed by patronising tolerance and finally complete absorption. Today, we can see manual therapy slotting into its rightful place in the treatment spectrum. It is up to the therapist to use it prudently, sparingly and within the limitations of his own individual competence.

This book does not pretend to compete with or imitate the many excellent works on the physiological and biomechanical theories of joint movement. It is simply an *aide-mémoire* for those who possess the appropriate professional qualifications and have undertaken suitable training.

The first edition was originally prepared as an illustrated companion for students attending the postgraduate course on joint mobilisation conducted by the Danish Physiotherapists' Manual Therapy Group. In response to repeated requests from the physiotherapy profession in Britain, we have added brief explanatory notes to the pictures. It is not possible to describe elegant, safe and effective techniques in mere words and pictures. The holds shown are starting positions for procedures whose dynamics can be understood only after adequate tuition and experience.

Various systems of gradation have been suggested to help in the prescription of manual treatments. The difficulty lies in the rigidity such a concept could impose. All techniques must be simple, so that they can be matched to the special requirements of each patient. The therapist must be a professional craftsman and not a mechanic turning out drill-like, stereotyped treatments.

TEACHING MANIPULATIVE TECHNIQUES

The practical difficulties of teaching techniques have been bedevilled by those who claim that manipulation is an art. Admittedly there are therapists whose ability and attainment raise them above the rest of us. Nevertheless, just because we cannot all be Rembrandts it does not mean that by following the instructions and painting carefully along the prescribed lines we cannot make a fair job of 'painting by numbers'. The numerous text-books depicting techniques by photograph and diagram should never be used for teaching; their function should be as *aides-mémoire*. There is no substitute for watching and learning the skills and attitudes from an experienced, expert and ethical clinician. Once the technique has been understood and mastered, the therapist must learn to adapt the basic patterns to his own requirements. Because there are no stereo-typed techniques, each treatment is different and belongs to the therapist and the patient at that particular time.

GENERAL CONSIDERATIONS

Position of the patient

Ensure that the following criteria are satisfied:
- the patient is comfortable and relaxed throughout the entire procedure
- in the sitting position it is essential that the patient is kept 'in balance'; this means that the occiput should be in line with the coccyx, thus keeping the apex above the base
- the joint under treatment is accessible and the full range of movement remains unrestricted
- it is essential that the movement can be localised to the exact area required.

Position of the therapist

While offering maximum support to the patient, the therapist must remember that he too has to be comfortable. There will be many other bodies to be looked after in the future. A particular technique that hurts or tires should be abandoned and another one found. Positions that offer maximum mechanical advantage should be devised and at the same time a relaxed and balanced stance maintained.

Grip

The grip must be firm and reassuring, while at the same time allowing the fingertips to be free to palpate the tissues under treatment. A weak grip is irritating, but a grip that is too firm induces reflex muscle spasm. There is a happy medium— find it. Often, a double-handed grip will give the stability and control required. There are many examples in this book.

Pain

There are very few circumstances which justify the infliction of pain. Properly executed, none of the techniques included in this book should hurt the patient.

CLASSIFICATION OF TECHNIQUES

The multitude of manual techniques at the disposal of the therapist can be divided into three broad categories:
- massage techniques
- passive articulatory movements
- procedures involving a thrust of high velocity.

Massage techniques

These include kneading, effleurage, stretching and springing. Probably because they are time-consuming and of unproven physiological value, these techniques have recently lost popularity. Nevertheless, they are of great value as introductory treatments. They help to familiarise the patient with the physiotherapist's touch, inducing confidence and relaxation. They also provide an opportunity for palpatory diagnosis.

Passive articulatory movements

These form the basis of most of the techniques depicted in this book. Their performance is slow, rhythmic and repetitive. The physiotherapist initiates and controls the movement while the patient complies with and follows the pattern— rather like the partner in a dance. Where possible, the therapist should allow his fingertips to be free from pressure in order to palpate and monitor the patient's tissues.

High velocity thrust

This is the most dramatic, most abused yet often the most effective tool the therapist possesses. High velocity thrust must never be allowed to degenerate to the status of a placebo, nor should it be undertaken lightly since occasional tragedies occur even in the hands of the professional manipulator. Should the therapist fail to achieve his objective with a thrust technique, he should never be tempted to 'have another go'. He should be wise and humble enough to recognise that the patient's protective reflexes have made a better estimation of the situation, and accept this conclusion with grace.

Mechanically, the technique is achieved by a combination of *leverage* and *thrust*. The function of leverage is to localise the movement to one specific joint. The thrust engenders kinetic energy, to produce a sheering effect which has enough velocity to forestall the natural protective reflex mechanism of the body.

The distinction between passive articulatory movements and high velocity thrust can be summarised as follows:

Passive movements	*High velocity thrust*
Slow, rhythmic and repetitive	Rapid 'single shot'
Patient participating	Patient relaxed
Within the elastic recoil of the patient's tissues	Pre-empts patient's protective reflexes
Generalised target	Localised target

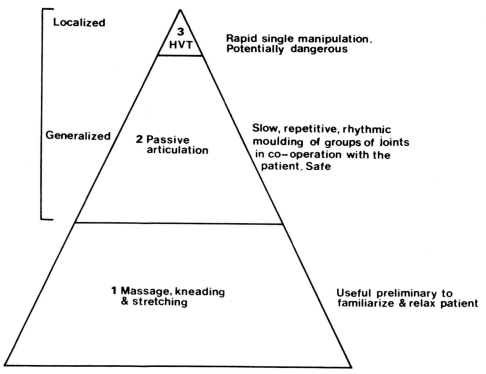

Fig. 1 Diagram depicting ascending scale of force. A scheme illustrating frequency of use of the three basic types of manual technique. (HVT = High velocity thrust.)

The manual therapist's options are depicted in Figure 1, with the available procedures arranged in an ascending scale of force. Additionally, the proportions represented by each of the headings indicate the frequency of their use.

BIOMECHANICS

All manual procedures are essentially a combination of two elements: leverage and thrust. Usually, these are applied in inverse proportion to each other. This concept can be depicted diagrammatically by a mathematical model consisting of a rectangle bisected diagonally, with one segment representing leverage and the other representing thrust (Fig. 2). Any line drawn vertically down through the model will pass through varying proportions of each element. Thus passive stretching could be placed on the extreme left of the diagram, at A–B, while the sudden chiropractic thrust will be on the right, at C–D. Most high velocity thrusts are a combination of both elements and would fall into the broad band E–F.

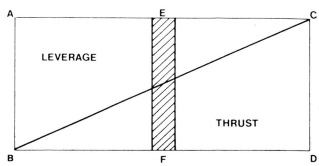

Fig. 2 Scheme to illustrate the combinations, in inverse proportion, of leverage and thrust in manual techniques

Properties of leverage	*Properties of thrust*
Length of lever arm	Velocity: acceleration & arrest
Amplitude	Plane or 90°
Traction or compression	Amplitude
Primary or secondary	Timing: early/late/synchronized

Properties of leverage

Length of lever arm

Obviously, the strength of the leverage is partially dependent upon the length of the lever and as a general rule this should be as short as is practical and comfortable.

Amplitude

This refers to the arc through which the lever is operated and is therefore related to the amount of movement the therapist wishes to impart to the joint. In some cases a long swinging amplitude helps to relax the patient.

Traction

It is often helpful to segregate the joint surfaces during manipulative procedures. But traction is no substitute for prudence and care. If you consider that a technique can only be made safe by traction, do not use it.

Compression

Occasionally the apposition of two adjacent surfaces will reduce the need for leverage.

Properties of thrust

Plane

The torsional forces imposed by the leverage must localise all available movement to one specific articulation. Therefore, when the thrust is delivered, its course can be directed along the plane of the facets of the target joint.

Amplitude

This refers to the distance the thrust is set to travel. Quite obviously, if the distance exceeds the normal articular range of the joint, substantial damage will result. As with so many activities in life, the trick is in knowing when and how to stop.

Timing

The thrust must be synchronised with the moment at which the forces of leverage culminate on the target joint.

Force

This has to be minimal. The greater the skill of the therapist the gentler he will become. The converse is dreadfully true.

It seems strange that, after so many years of use, no adequate explanation has been found for the biomechanics of the high velocity thrust. Figure 3 shows that there are many ways in which object A can be moved in relation to object B.

All manual treatments are displacing the tissues against the body's own inertia.

What is doing the displacing? It is force, and

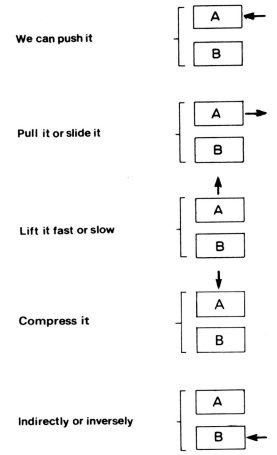

Fig. 3 The variety of ways in which one body may be moved in relation to an adjacent one

because this force is potentially dangerous, we must consider its properties. Force is defined as the effect one body has upon another . It is a vector quantity, with magnitude and direction. It is the latter factor that principally concerns us, because unless force is directed accurately, the procedure is not only useless but is also hazardous.

Velocity

Obviously the difference between passive articulation and high velocity thrust is *velocity*.

Velocity is defined as the rate of displacement. It is directly proportional to the length of displacement and inversely proportional to the time taken. This can be represented:

$$\text{Velocity} = \frac{\text{Distance}}{\text{Time}}$$

Acceleration

Now a new factor enters our equation — acceleration is defined as the rate of change in velocity. Newton's Second Law declares that the acceleration of an object is directly proportional to the force applied, in the same direction as that force and inversely proportional to the mass. So we get the equation:

$$Acceleration (A) = \frac{Force\ (F)}{Mass\ (M)}$$

$$A = \frac{F}{M}$$

Which resolves

$$F = M \times A$$

Now consider a time-honoured analogy (Fig. 4). To drive a hefty wooden stake into the ground, we could use either a sledge-hammer or a bullet fired from a pistol. The sledge-hammer would represent a large mass with slow acceleration, which would slowly pound the stake into the earth. The bullet would represent a small mass with tremendous acceleration; the force imparted to the stake would culminate more rapidly than the structure of the wood could absorb and the stake would shatter. The sledge-

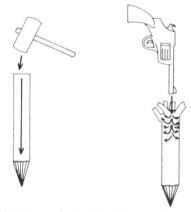

Fig. 4 Scheme to symbolise the difference between effects of low velocity passive movement and the high velocity thrust

hammer represents passive movement whereas the bullet is analagous to the high velocity thrust.

CONTRA-INDICATIONS

While it is obvious that caution should be exercised at all times, there are circumstances in which these techniques of manipulation should either be modified or avoided altogether:

1. Where the structure of the bone has been weakened by pathological processes including neoplastic change, inflammation or severe osteoporosis
2. Where there are symptoms derived from severe radicular or cauda equina pressure
3. Where the integrity of ligaments may be affected by the use of steroids. This applies especially to the upper cervical area
4. Where vertebral artery insufficiency is suspected
5. Where it is instinctively felt that manual treatment would be traumatic.

If in doubt ... don't!

CONCLUSION

The added dimension of manipulation in physical therapy requires discretion, initiative and manual ability. Although manual therapists are privileged to exercise skills which can give great job satisfaction, they also undertake responsibilities. It is only by a recognition of personal limitations that we can ensure the safety of patients and bring credit to our craft.

IMPORTANT NOTE

The following note applies to the Plate illustrations that appear throughout the rest of the book:

Arrow   represents the direction of pressure or of movement.

Cross   represents a fixed point.

There is no significance in the colour or size of the arrows.

THE CERVICAL SPINE

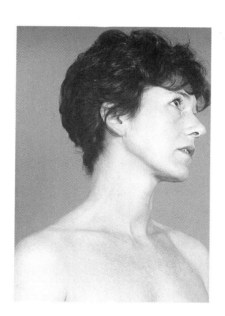
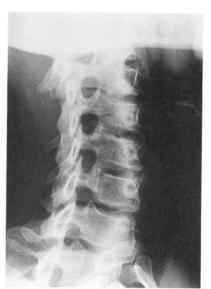
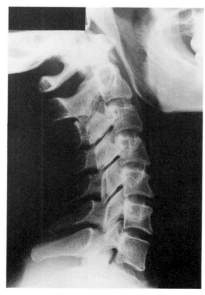
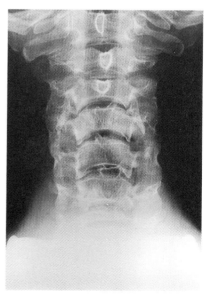

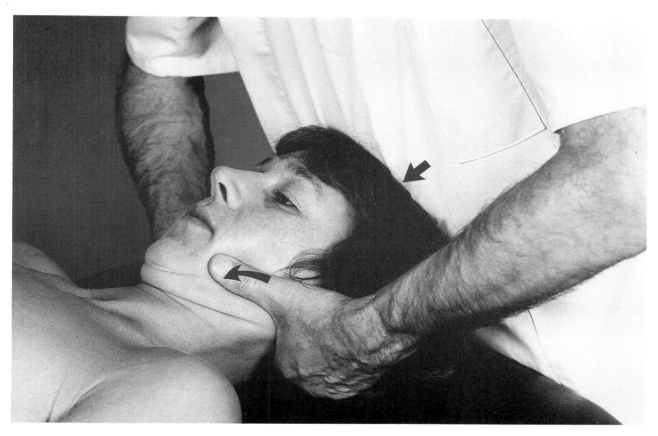

Plate 1
CERVICAL FLEXION

Patient	Lying supine.
Operator	Standing at the head of the plinth.
Technique	The operator stabilises the patient's head with his abdomen, and by depressing the rami of the patient's mandible with his thumbs produces flexion of the cervical spine.

THE CERVICAL SPINE

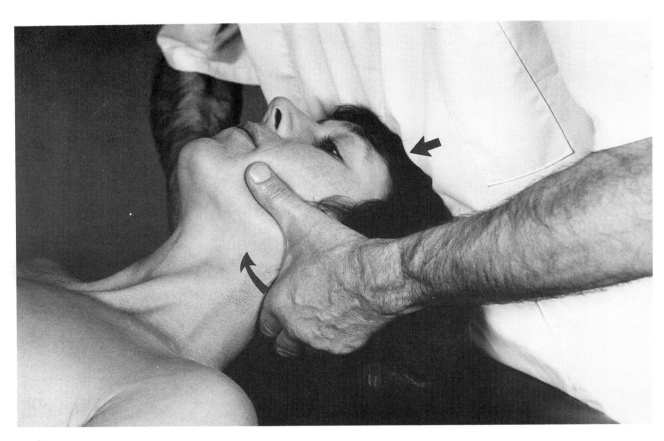

Plate 2
CERVICAL EXTENSION

Patient	Lying supine.
Operator	Standing at the head of the plinth.
Technique	The operator stabilises the patient's head with his abdomen. Extension is produced by lifting the posterior aspect of each vertebral level with the index fingers of both hands simultaneously.

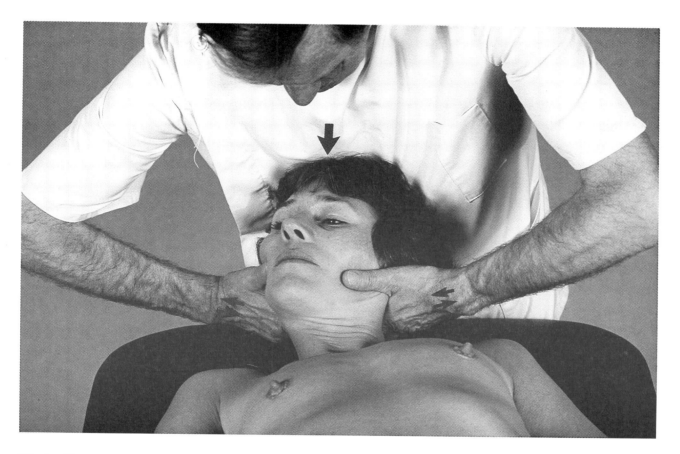

Plate 3
CERVICAL SIDE FLEXION

Patient	Lying supine.
Operator	Standing at the head of the plinth.
Technique	The operator stabilises the patient's head with his abdomen. Side flexion is obtained by the application of lateral pressure to the appropriate vertebral level with the metacarpophalangeal joints of the index fingers. The wrists must be held straight to ensure an accurate line to the articular surface.

THE CERVICAL SPINE

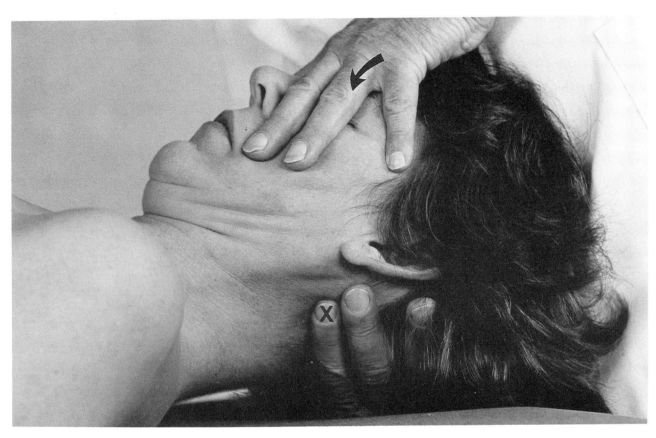

Plate 4
ATLANTO-OCCIPITAL ARTICULATION

Patient	Lying supine.
Operator	Standing at the head of the plinth.
Technique	The patient's head is supported between the palms of the operator's hands. The fingers of the upper hand are spread over the forehead and maxillae, while the pads of the thumb and index finger of the lower hand grasp the posterior arches of the atlas. Springing of the atlanto-occipital joint is effected by downwards pressure from the upper hand.

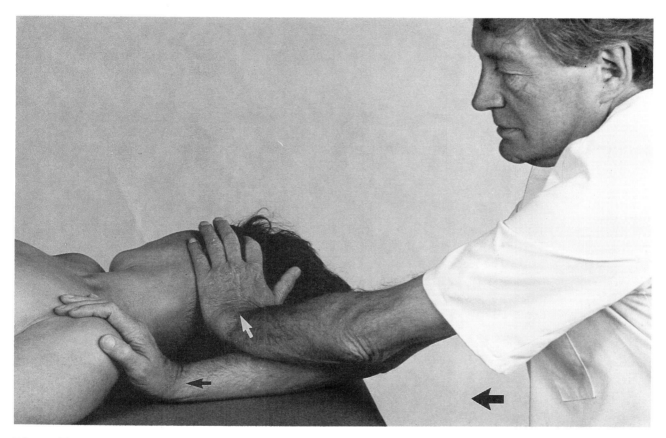

Plate 5
CERVICAL SIDE STRETCHING

Patient	Lying supine.
Operator	Standing at the head of the plinth.
Technique	Here the crossed arms of the operator act like the blades of a pair of scissors which separate as he brings his body forward towards the patient, thus stretching the cervical spine.

THE CERVICAL SPINE

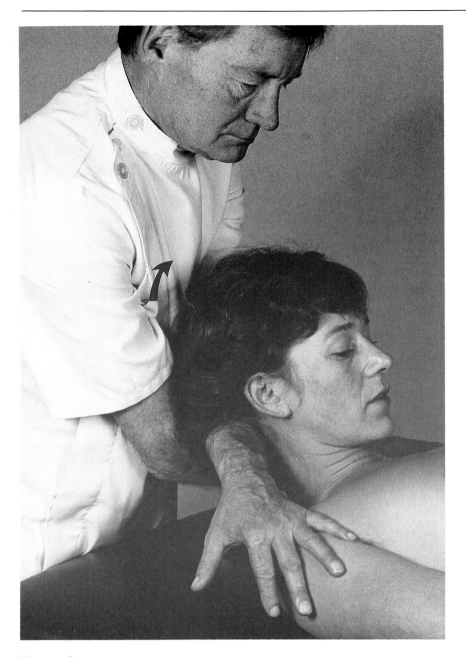

Plate 6
CERVICAL STRETCHING IN FLEXION

Patient   Lying supine.

Operator   Standing at the head of the plinth.

Technique   The crossed arms of the operator form a cradle for the patient's head. By
              rising on his toes, the operator stretches the neck into flexion.

THE CERVICAL SPINE

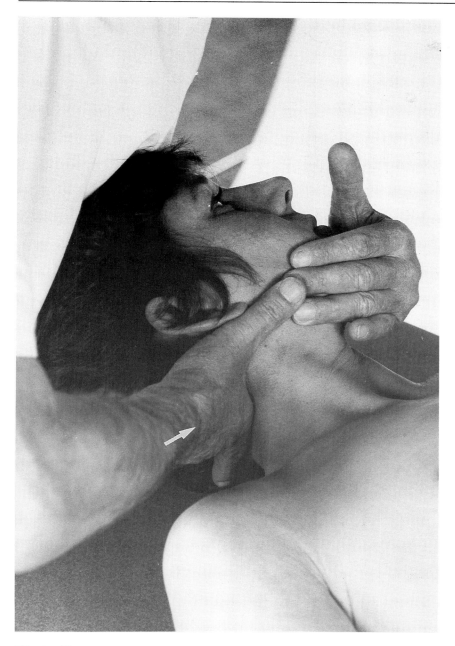

Plate 7
MOBILISATION OF THE CERVICAL SPINE

Patient   Lying supine.

Operator   Standing at the head of the plinth.

Technique   With one hand, forearm and pectoral area the operator forms a cradle for
              the patient's head. The other hand acts as an applicator, with the
              metacarpophalangeal joint of the index finger pressed against the
              appropriate articular pillar.

THE CERVICAL SPINE

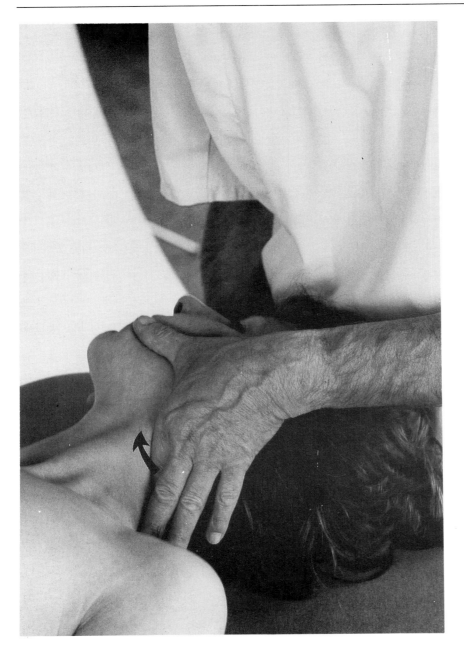

Plate 8
MOBILISATION OF THE CERVICAL SPINE

Patient   Lying supine.

Operator   Standing at the head of the plinth.

Technique   While one of the operator's hands supports the weight of the patient's head, the other hand obtains rotation. The contact point is the appropriate articular pillar, and the applicator is the metacarpophalangeal joint of the index finger.

THE CERVICAL SPINE

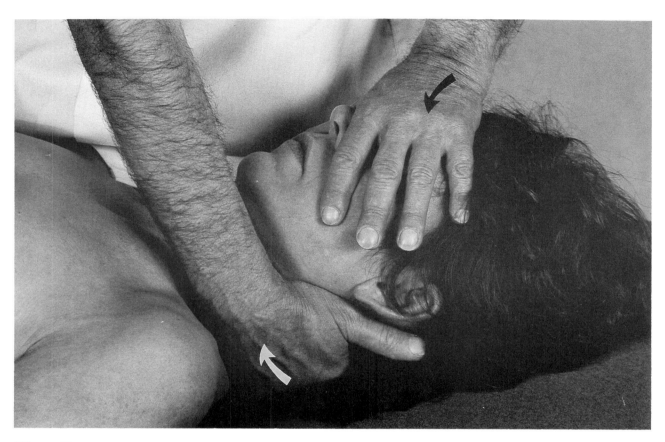

Plate 9
GENERAL MOBILISATION OF THE CERVICAL SPINE

Patient	Lying supine.
Operator	Standing at the side of the plinth.
Technique	The spread fingers of the operator's left hand stabilise the patient's head, while the fingers of the right hand lift and roll the cervical spine. Both hands work in diametric opposition to each other, to effect full range of cervical movement.

THE CERVICAL SPINE

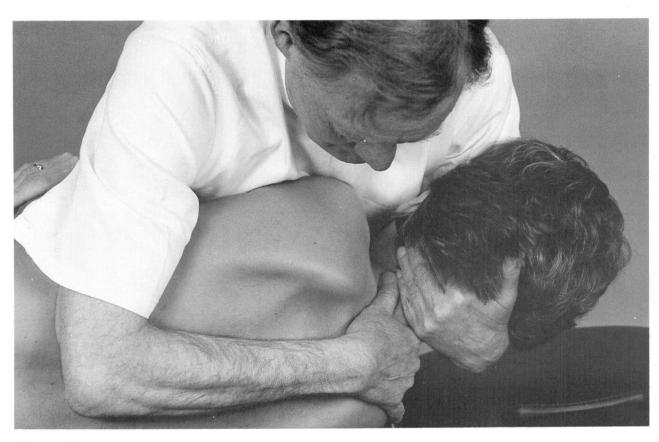

Plate 10
MOBILISATION OF THE CERVICAL SPINE IN SIDE LYING

Patient   Side lying, facing the operator.

Operator   Standing at the side of the plinth.

Technique   The patient's head is supported in the operator's left hand, while the right hand and arm stabilise the thorax. By keeping the two hands in close apposition, localised and controlled cervical movements can be obtained in all directions.

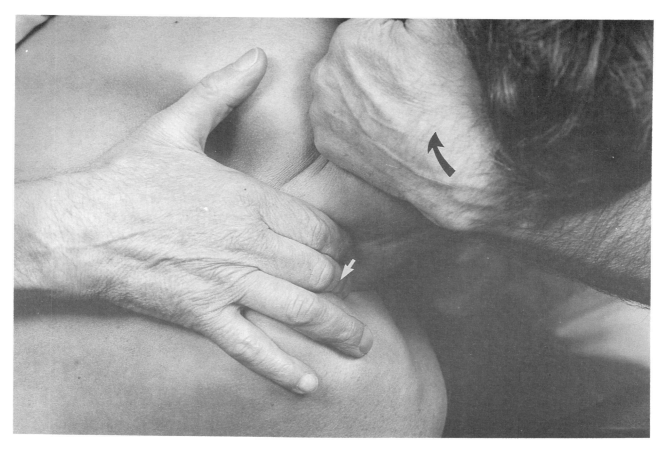

Plate 11
MOBILISATION OF THE FIRST RIB

Patient	Side lying, facing the operator.
Operator	Standing at the side of the plinth.
Technique	The patient's head is supported in the operator's left hand, while the index and middle fingers of the right hand hook around the first rib. Mobilisation of the first costothoracic joint is effected by side flexion and counter rotation of the patient's neck and head.

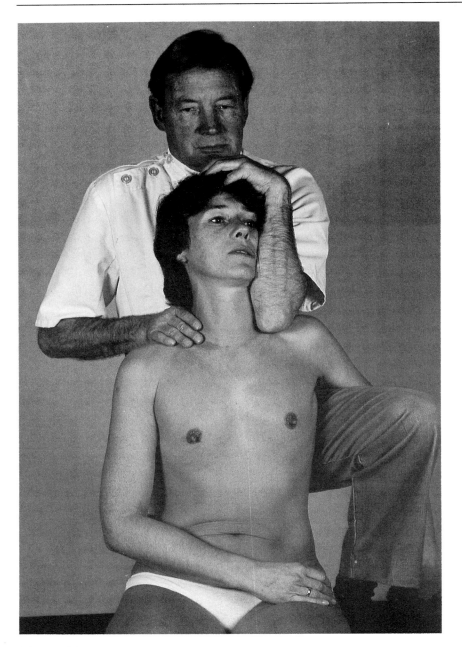

Plate 12
MOBILISATION OF THE CERVICOTHORACIC AREA

Patient   Sitting.

Operator   Standing behind the patient with his left thigh under her axilla and his body supporting her weight.

Technique With the left hand and forearm stabilising the patient's head and neck, and maintaining the head in line with the sacrum, the right hand forms a fulcrum around which movements are produced and directed.

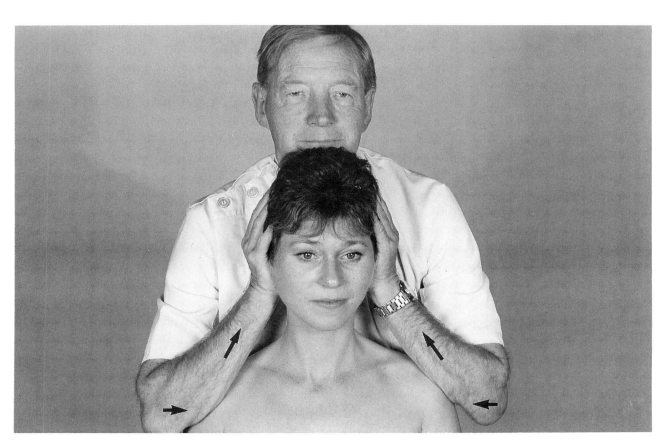

Plate 13
TRACTION TO THE CERVICAL SPINE

Patient	Sitting.
Operator	Standing behind the patient.
Technique	The operator's forearms form two sides of a triangle, with the palms of his hands at its apex. By bringing his elbows towards each other, the base of the triangle is shortened, thus producing traction in the cervical spine.

THE CERVICAL SPINE

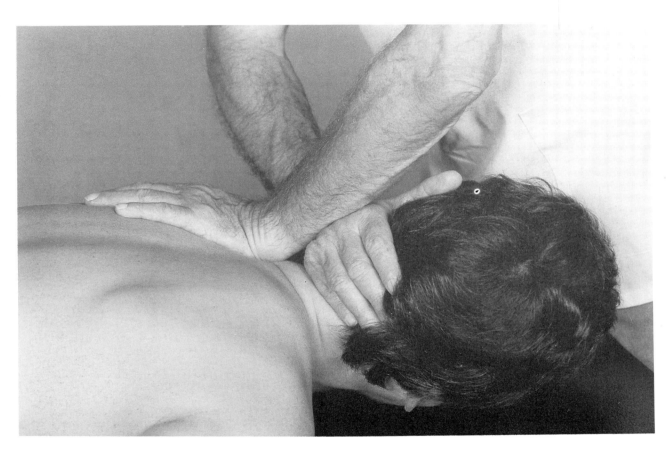

Plate 14
MOBILISATION OF THE CERVICOTHORACIC JUNCTION

Patient	Prone lying with the head pivoting on the chin.
Operator	Standing at the head of the plinth.
Technique	While the operator cups the patient's occiput with one hand, his other hand exerts pressure on the suprascapular region, thus stretching and mobilising the cervicothoracic junction.

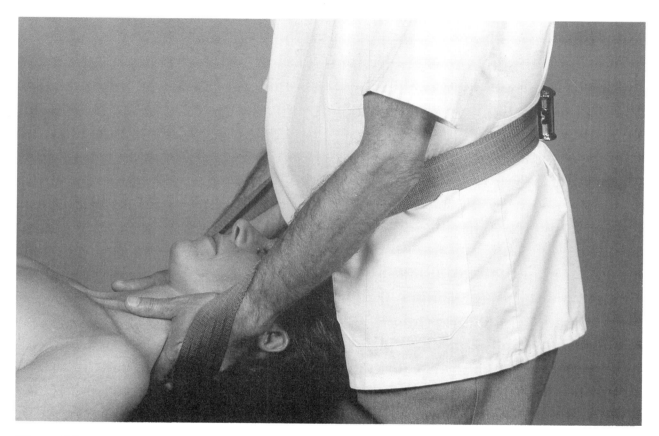

Plate 15

TRACTION TO THE CERVICAL SPINE USING A STRAP

Patient	Lying supine.
Operator	Standing at the head of the plinth.
Technique	The strap encircles the operator's body and hands but it should not come into contact with the patient's neck. By leaning backwards, the operator produces tension in the strap which is transmitted through his hands to the patient's cervical spine.

THE
THORACIC
SPINE

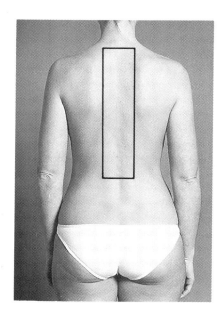
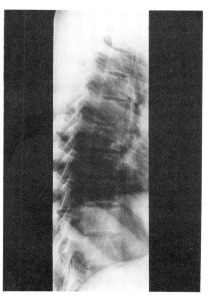
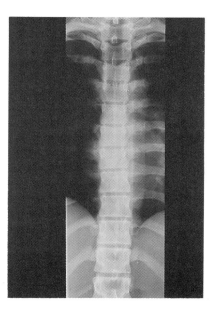

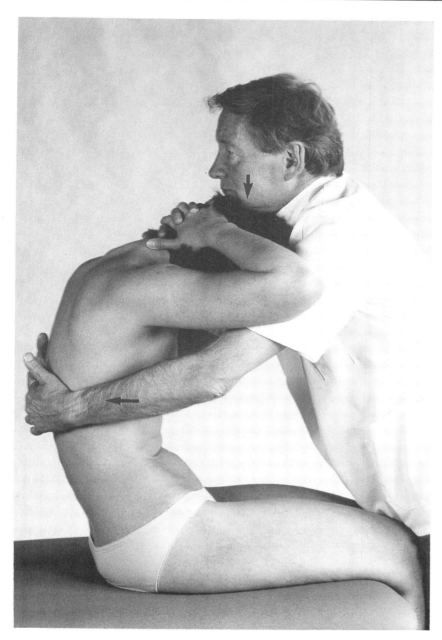

Plate 16
FLEXION OF THE THORACIC SPINE

Patient	Sitting facing the operator, with hands clasped behind her neck.
Operator	Standing and grasping the patient's thighs between his knees, and with his arms around the thorax.
Technique	By pressing down upon the vertex of the patient's head with his chin, the operator obtains a full range of flexion. His fingers palpate and monitor the movement.

THE THORACIC SPINE

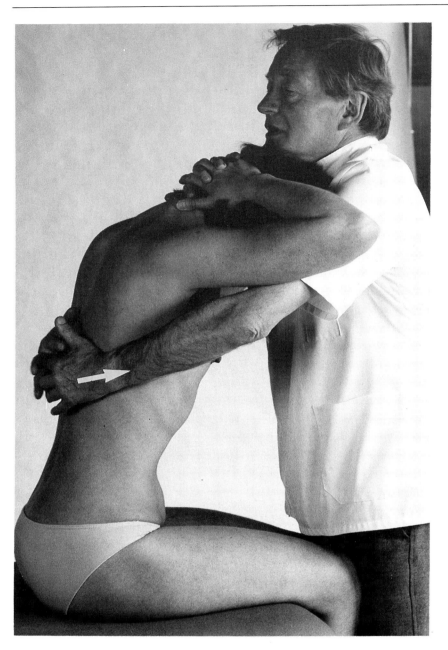

Plate 17
EXTENSION OF THE THORACIC SPINE

Patient   Sitting facing the operator, with hands clasped behind her neck.

Operator   Standing and grasping the patient's thighs between his knees, and with his arms around the thorax.

Technique While his fingers palpate and monitor the movement, the operator draws the patient's thoracic spine towards him.

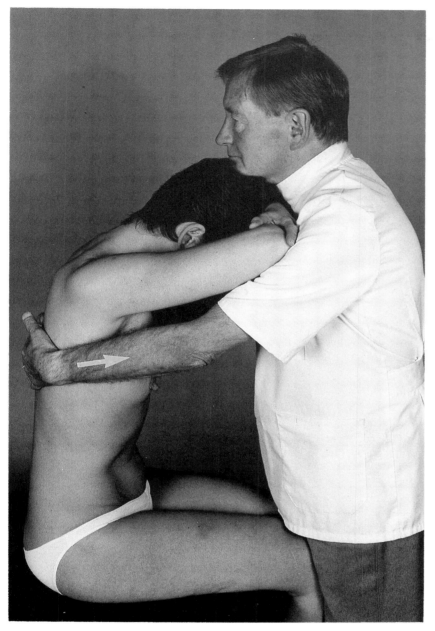

Plate 18
EXTENSION OF THE THORACIC SPINE

Patient	Sitting facing the operator, with her arms folded in front of her and resting on the operator.
Operator	Standing grasping the patient's thighs between his knees, and with his arms around the thorax.
Technique	While his fingers palpate and monitor the movement, the operator draws the patient's thoracic spine towards him.

THE THORACIC SPINE

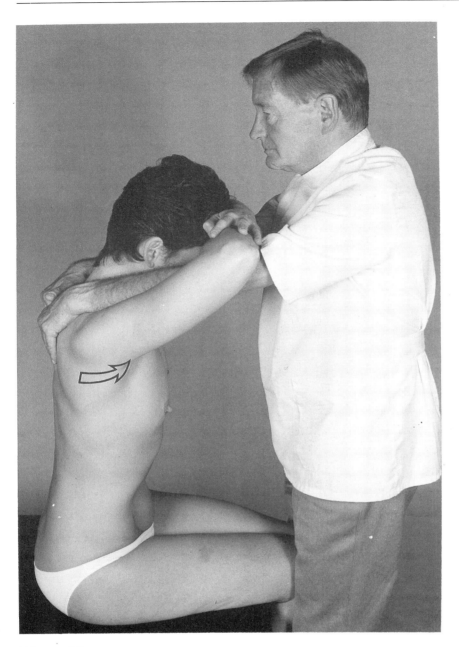

Plate 19
EXTENSION OF THE THORACIC SPINE

Patient	Sitting facing the operator, with arms folded in front of her.
Operator	Standing grasping the patient's thighs between his knees.
Technique	With his arms threaded through the patient's folded arms and with his fingers palpating the interscapular area, the operator draws the patient towards him, producing extension in the upper thoracic spine.

THE THORACIC SPINE

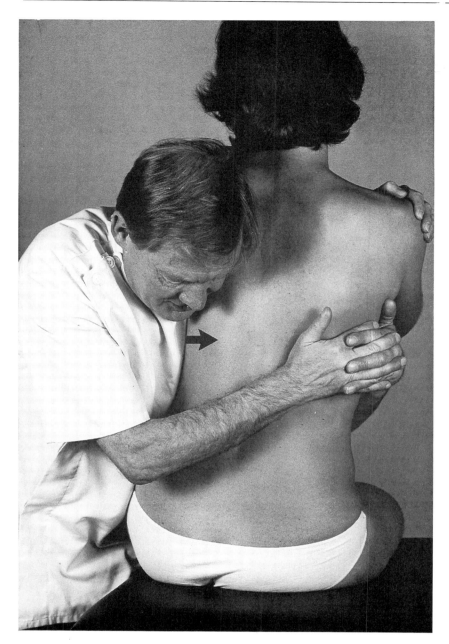

Plate 20
SIDE BENDING OF THE THORACIC SPINE TO THE LEFT

Patient	Sitting at the end of the plinth with legs over one side and arms clasped across her chest.
Operator	Standing at the foot of the plinth, with his fingers interlocked around the thorax.
Technique	Using his shoulder as a fulcrum, the operator leans forward thus side bending the patient's spine to the left, keeping her head in line with the sacrum.

THE THORACIC SPINE

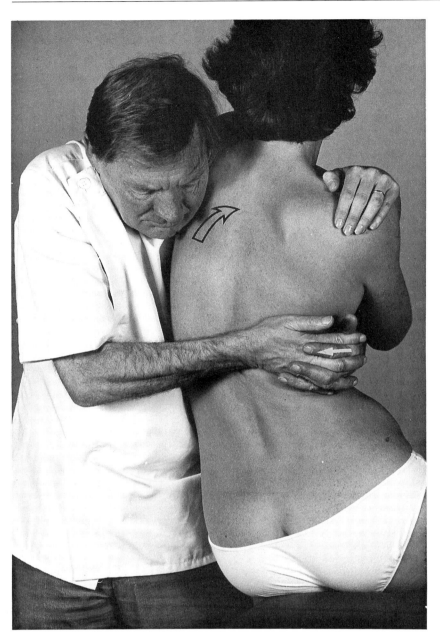

Plate 21
SIDE BENDING OF THE THORACIC SPINE TO THE RIGHT

Patient   Sitting at the end of the plinth with legs over one side and arms clasped across her chest.

Operator   Standing at the foot of the plinth.

Technique With his interlocked fingers, the operator draws the patient's thorax towards him, while at the same time raising his shoulder to lift the patient's axilla. The patient's head should remain vertically above her sacrum.

THE THORACIC SPINE

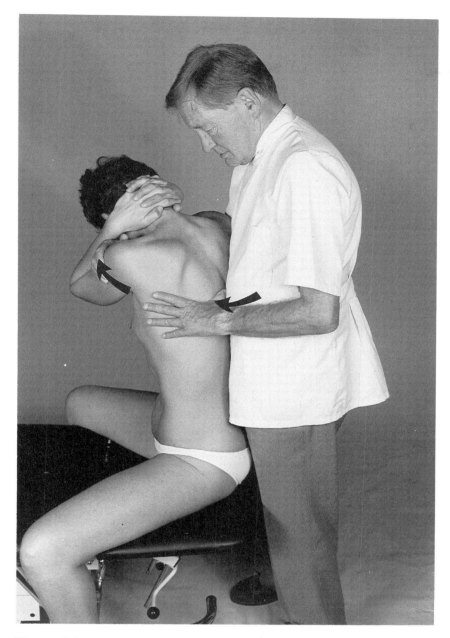

Plate 22
ROTATION OF THE THORACIC SPINE

Patient	Sitting astride the plinth with arms clasped behind her neck.
Operator	Standing behind the patient.
Technique	Threading his right arm through the patient's flexed arms and grasping her shoulder, the operator moves his whole body to effect rotation, while his free hand controls and augments the movement.

THE THORACIC SPINE

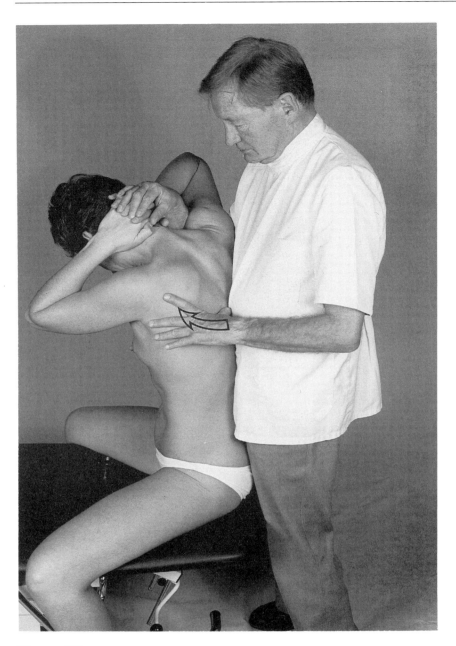

Plate 23
ROTATION OF THE THORACIC SPINE (ALTERNATIVE HOLD)

Patient	Sitting astride the plinth with arms clasped behind her neck.
Operator	Standing behind the patient.
Technique	Threading his right hand through the patient's flexed right arm, the operator grasps her clasped hands and then moves his body to effect rotation. His left hand augments and localises the movement.

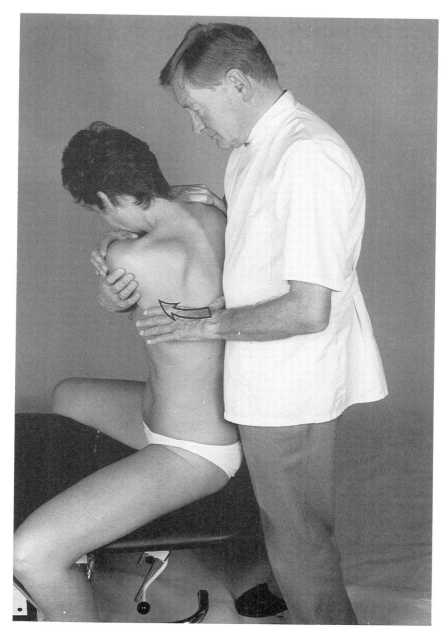

Plate 24
ROTATION OF THE THORACIC SPINE (ALTERNATIVE HOLD)

Patient	Sitting astride the plinth with arms clasped across her chest.
Operator	Standing at the foot of the plinth with his right arm threaded through the patient's folded arms to grasp her left shoulder.
Technique	Rotation of the spine is effected by the operator rotating the whole of his body and at the same time augmenting and localising the movement with his left hand.

THE THORACIC SPINE

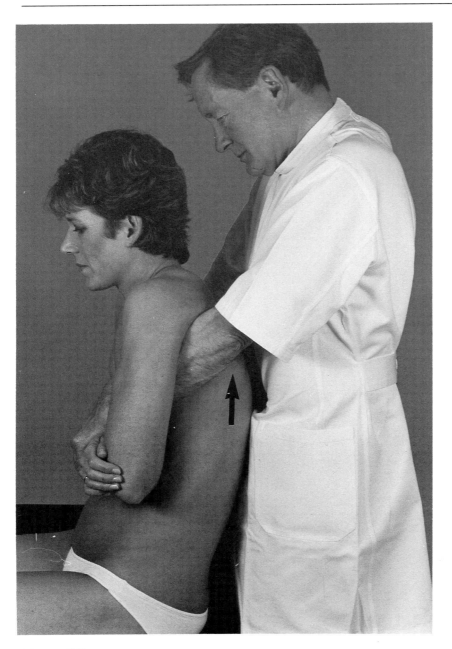

Plate 25
TRACTION TO THE THORACIC SPINE

Patient	Sitting, with arms folded in front of her thorax.
Operator	Grasping the patient's forearms with both hands and bringing her back towards his body.
Technique	The operator leans backwards to effect traction. Some degree of localisation can be obtained by varying the angle of flexion.

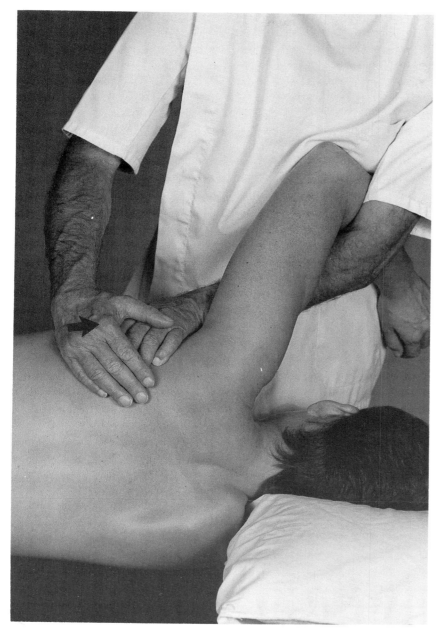

Plate 26
INTERCOSTAL STRETCHING (WITH RESPIRATION)

Patient   Side lying, with her left arm cradled by the operator's left arm.

Operator   Standing at the side of the plinth.

Technique   By pressing the ulnar border of his right hand into the intercostal space, the operator restricts the movement of the upper of the two ribs. The patient is then instructed to breathe in and out, thus allowing the thoracic excursion to separate the two adjacent ribs on expiration.

THE THORACIC SPINE

THE THORACIC SPINE

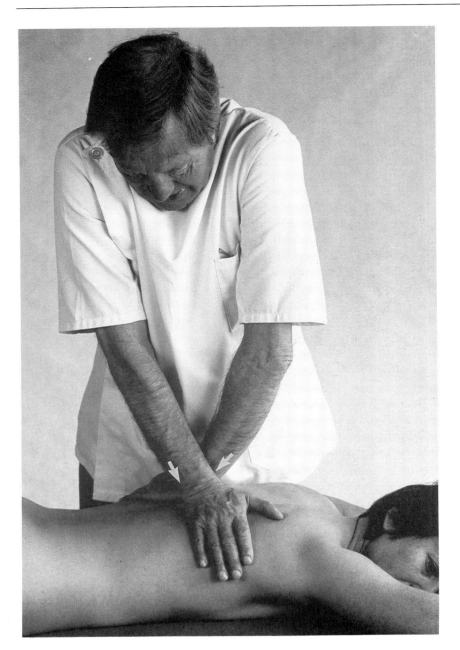

Plate 27
CROSS-HANDED SPRINGING OF THE THORAX (WITH RESPIRATION)

Patient   Lying prone.

Operator   Standing at the side of the plinth.

Technique With the pisiforms of both hands pressed firmly onto the transverse processes of a selected thoracic vertebra, gentle pressure is applied by the operator rising on his toes and then slowly descending onto his heels. The pressure is synchronised with expiration.

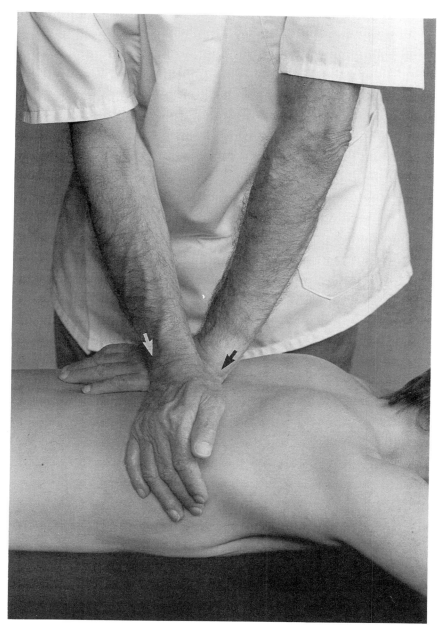

Plate 28
MOBILISATION OF INDIVIDUAL RIBS

Patient	Lying prone.
Operator	Standing at the side of the plinth.
Technique	The pisiform of the left hand is placed on the costotransverse area, while the pisiform of the right hand is placed below the angle of the same rib. Pressure is applied as the patient breathes out, in order to mobilise the costovertebral articulations.

THE THORACIC SPINE

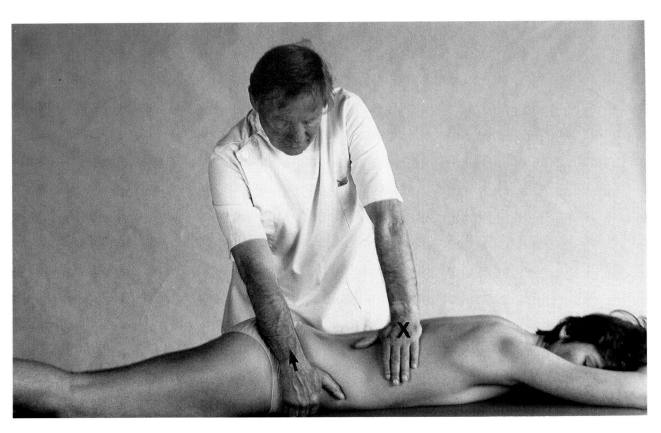

Plate 29
THORACIC MOBILISATION WITH LUMBAR LEVERAGE

Patient	Lying prone.
Operator	Standing beside the plinth.
Technique	The operator's right hand raises the anterior superior iliac spine, while his left hand fixes the thoracic spine at the appropriate level.

THE THORACIC SPINE

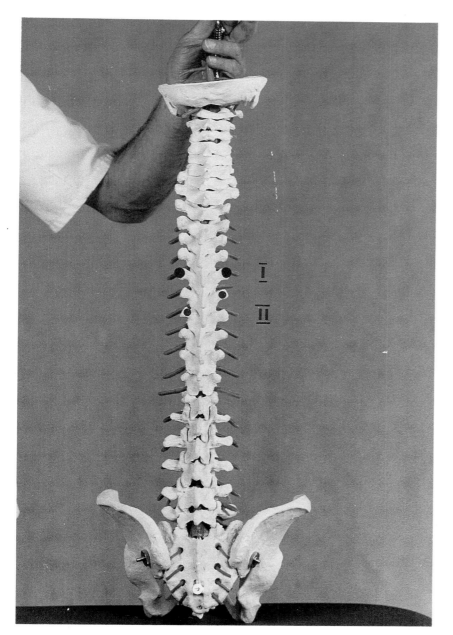

Plate 30
CONTACT POINTS FOR THRUST TECHNIQUES FOR THE THORACIC SPINE

The dots indicate the contact points for the techniques depicted in the following four plates. I, the transverse processes of the same vertebra; and II, the transverse processes of two adjacent vertebrae.

THE THORACIC SPINE

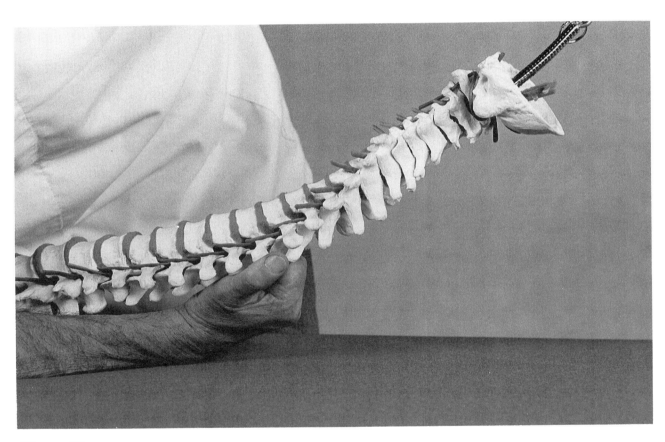

Plate 31
POSITION OF THE APPLICATOR FOR THRUST TECHNIQUES FOR THE
THORACIC SPINE

The applicator is the dorsal surface of the flexed middle phalanx of the index finger and
the base of the thumb of the operator's lower hand.

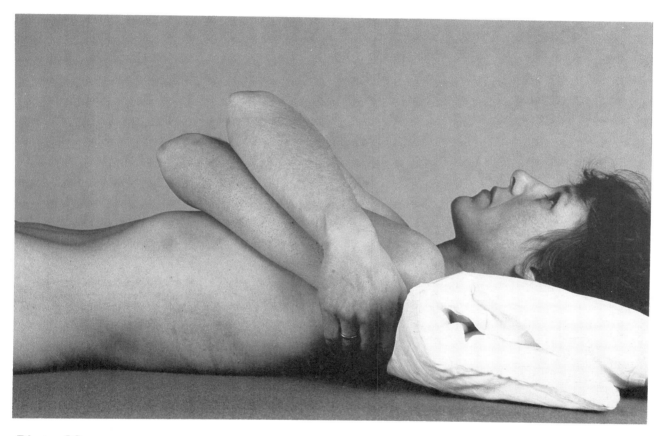

Plate 32

Patient's position for thrust techniques in the thoracic spine.

THE THORACIC SPINE

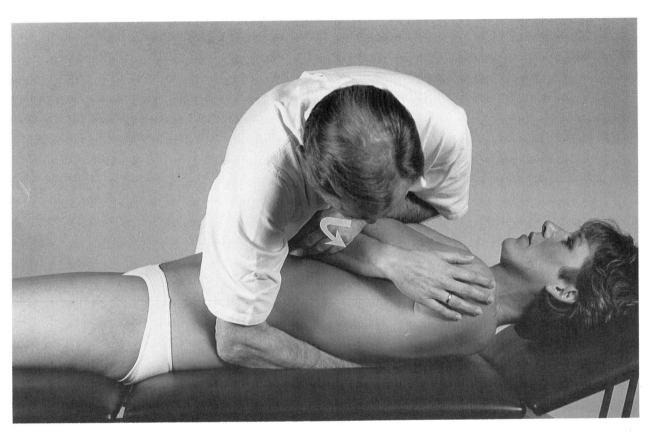

Plate 33
THRUST TECHNIQUES FOR THE THORACIC SPINE

Patient   Lying supine with arms folded across her chest.

Technique   Having placed the applicator accurately onto the contact points, the operator rolls the patient onto her back and applies an overpressure along the axes of the humeri, thus compressing the thorax onto the applicator. It is essential that the overpressure, or 'thrust', is synchronised with expiration.

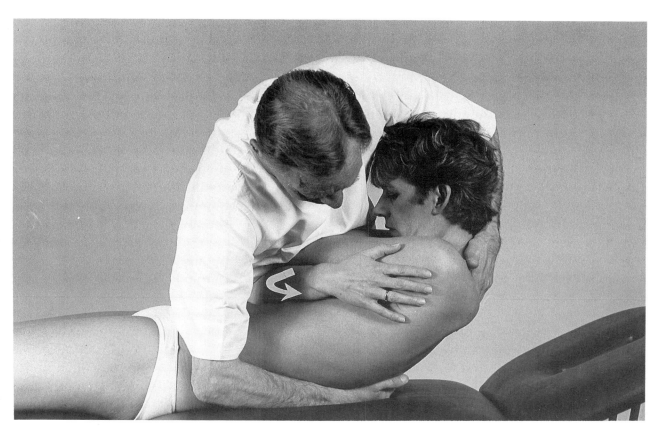

Plate 34

ALTERNATIVE HOLD FOR THRUST TECHNIQUES FOR THE LOWER
THORACIC SPINE

Here the operator adopts a hold around the patient's head and cervical region with his
left hand, and applies a thrust along the axes of the humeri with his epigastrium. The
thrust is synchronised with expiration.

THE LUMBAR SPINE

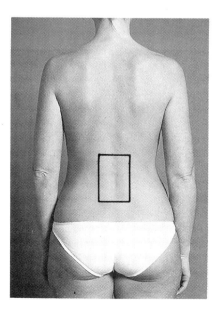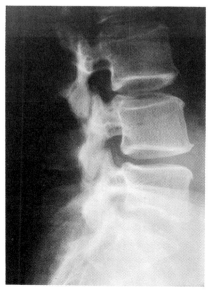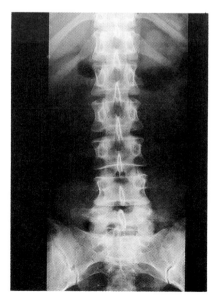

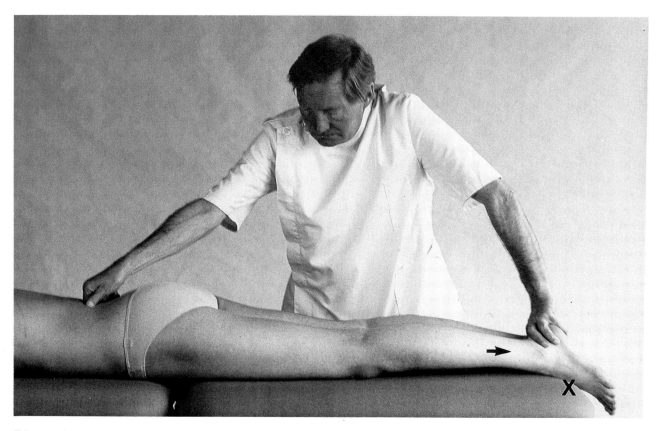

Plate 35
PRONE TRACTION TO THE LUMBAR SPINE

Patient	Lying prone, with the dorsum of both feet over the end of the plinth.
Operator	Standing at the side of the plinth.
Technique	While the operator palpates the lumbar spine with his right hand, he engenders a rocking motion by rhythmic pressure on the patient's heels; the dorsum of the patient's feet act as levers over the fulcrum provided by the edge of the plinth.

THE LUMBAR SPINE

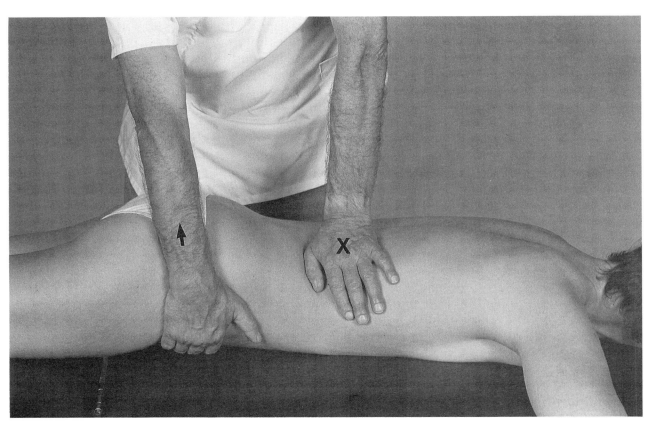

Plate 36
ROTATION OF THE LUMBAR SPINE

Patient	Lying prone.
Operator	Standing at the side of the plinth.
Technique	The operator's right hand raises the patient's anterior superior spine, while the left hand restricts the rotation to the selected vertebral level.

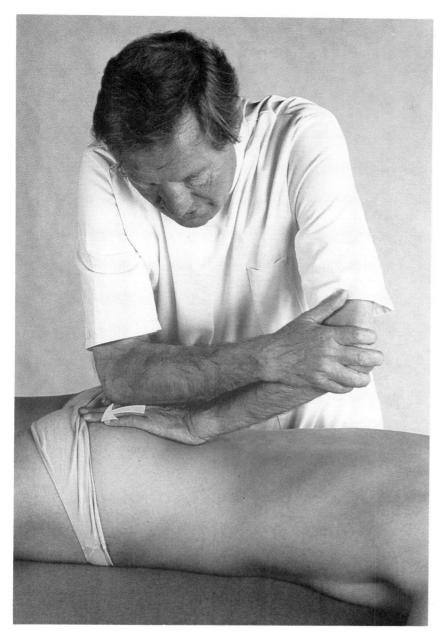

Plate 37
LUMBOSACRAL STRETCHING

THE LUMBAR SPINE

Patient	Lying prone.
Operator	Standing at the side of the plinth.
Technique	The operator's left hand is placed upon the sacrum with the elbow of his right arm resting between the index and middle fingers. By transferring his weight towards the foot of the plinth, a downward and caudal pressure is exerted on the sacrum.

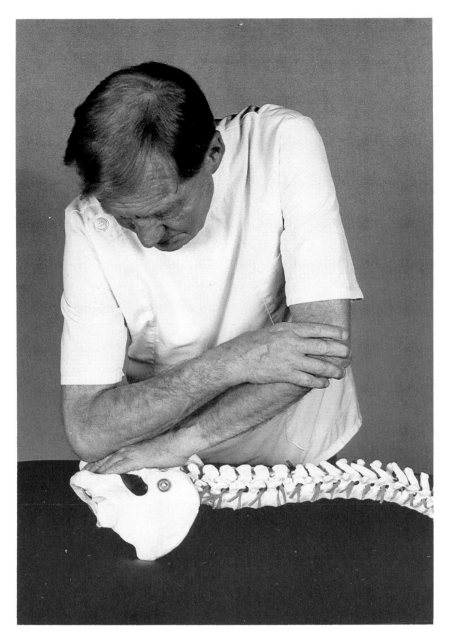

Plate 38
LUMBOSACRAL STRETCHING

Demonstration of the hold in relation to the skeleton.

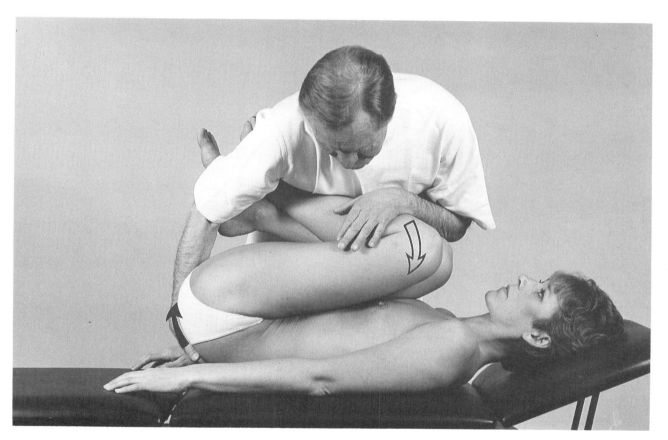

Plate 39
SUPINE FLEXION OF THE LUMBAR SPINE

Patient   Lying supine.

Operator   Standing at the side of the plinth.

Technique   The operator places his hand underneath the patient's sacrum. By transferring his weight towards the patient's head, flexion is produced in the lumbar spine. The left arm is supporting the patient's legs and augmenting the movement.

THE LUMBAR SPINE

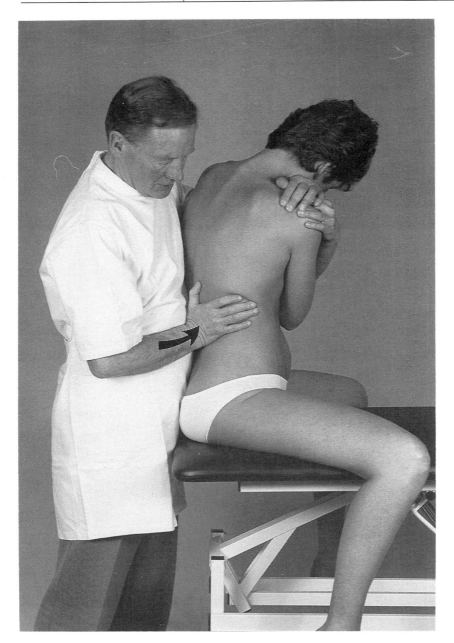

Plate 40
ROTATION OF THE LUMBAR SPINE

Patient   Sitting astride the end of the plinth, with folded arms.

Operator   Standing behind the patient.

Technique Threading his left hand through the patient's arms and grasping her right shoulder, the operator moves his whole body to effect rotation. His right hand controls and augments the movement.

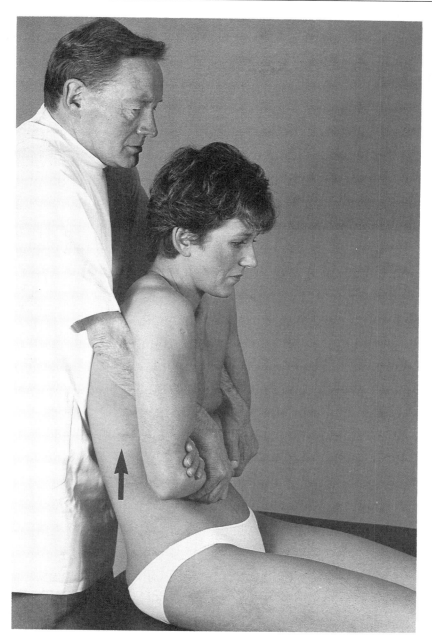

Plate 41
VERTICAL LIFT TO THE LUMBAR SPINE

Patient	Sitting relaxed against the operator.
Operator	Standing behind the patient.
Technique	The patient sits with arms folded across her chest. The operator grasps her forearms and, by rising on his toes, effects traction in her lumbar spine.

THE LUMBAR SPINE

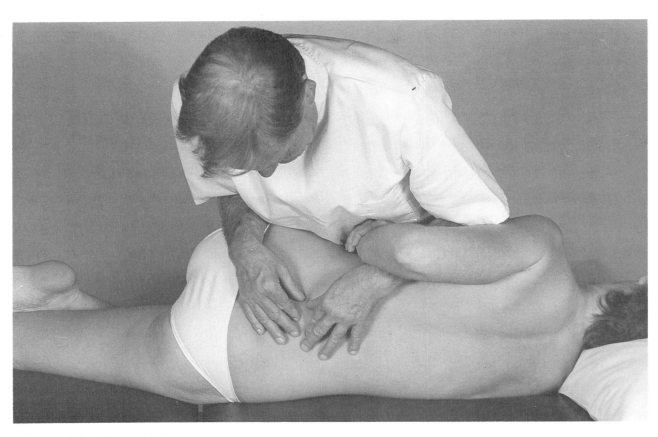

Plates 42, 43 and 44
HIGH VELOCITY THRUST OF THE LUMBAR SPINE

Patient   Side lying with the flexed upper knee clear of the plinth and the foot
             resting behind the straight lower leg.

Operator   Standing at the side of the plinth.

THE LUMBAR SPINE

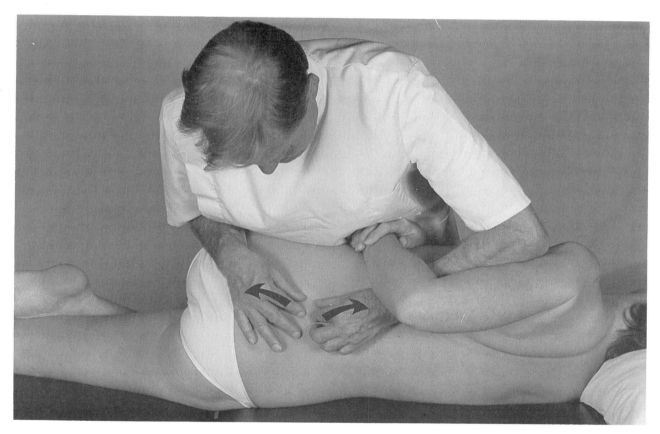

Plate 43

HIGH VELOCITY THRUST OF THE LUMBAR SPINE WITH TRACTION

Technique   The patient's lower arm is drawn forward to effect torsion in the thorax, which forms the upper lever. The pelvis is then rotated towards the operator, producing a counter torsion. This localises the movement to one selected segment of the lumbar spine. The thrust is a gentle overpressure applied by the operator's body weight through the flexor surface of his right forearm and abdomen to the patient's gluteal area. No pressure is applied to the patient's shoulder, which simply stabilises the upper lever. The operator's fingers should be free to palpate the tissues and augment the movement. A slight shift of the operator's stance will add either traction (Plate 43) or compression (Plate 44) to the articular surfaces.

THE LUMBAR SPINE

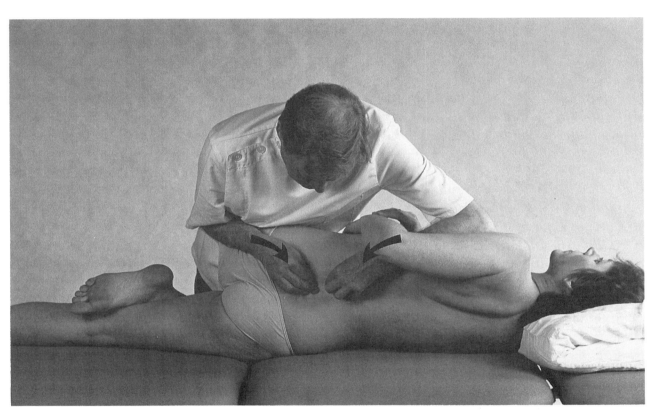

Plate 44
HIGH VELOCITY THRUST OF THE LUMBAR SPINE WITH COMPRESSION

SACRO-ILIAC JOINT

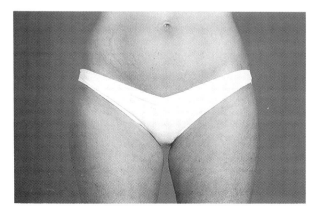 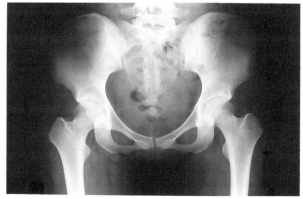

SACRO-ILIAC JOINT

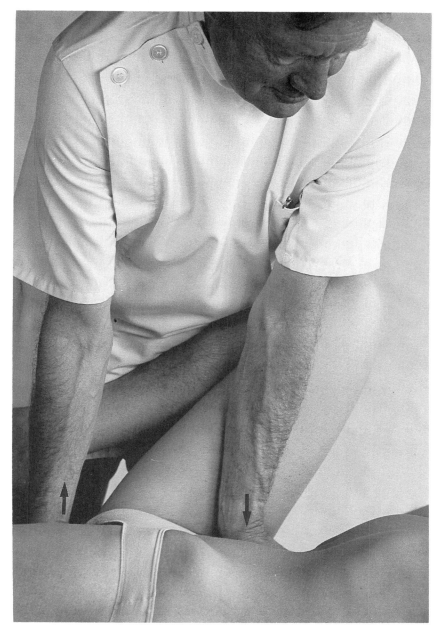

Plate 45
MOBILISATION OF THE SACRO-ILIAC JOINT

Patient ·	Lying supine.
Operator	Standing at the side of the plinth.
Principle	Assume the right ilium to be located in a position relatively anterior to the sacrum at the sacro-iliac joint.
Technique	The operator grasps the ischial tuberosity with his right hand and cups the anterior superior iliac spine in the palm of his left hand. Movement in the joint is obtained by the operator transferring his weight towards the patient's head.

SACRO-ILIAC JOINT

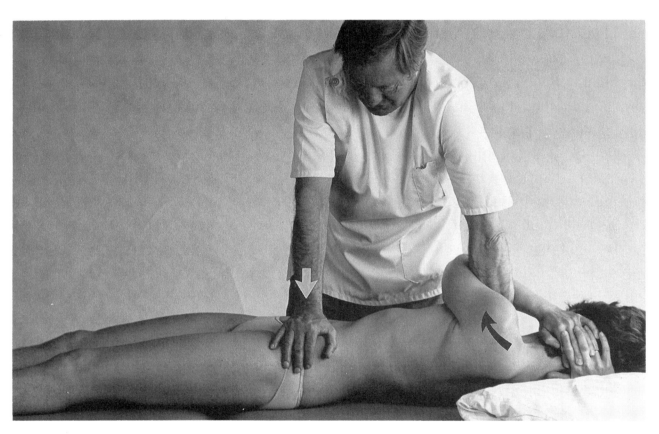

Plate 46
MOBILISATION OF THE SACRO-ILIAC JOINT

Patient	Lying supine in side bending, with the convexity of the curve towards the operator. Her hands are clasped behind her neck.
Operator	Standing at the side of the plinth.
Principle	Assume the left ilium to be located in a position relatively anterior to the sacrum at the sacro-iliac joint.
Technique	While the palm of his right hand cups the anterior superior iliac spine, the left hand is threaded through the patient's arms. The operator rotates the patient's thorax forward, while restraining movement at the level of the pelvis by pressure from his right hand.

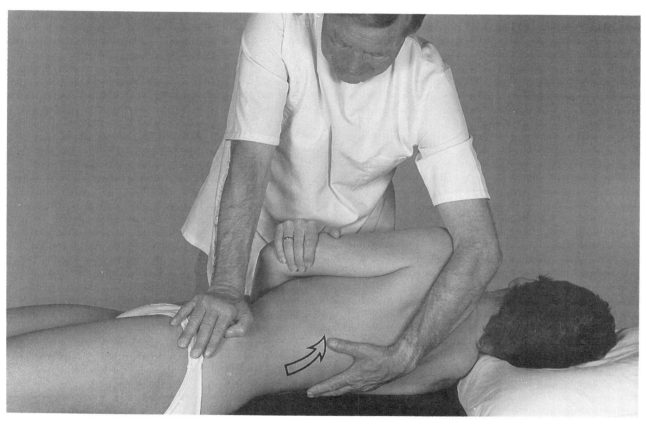

Plate 47
MOBILISATION OF THE SACRO-ILIAC JOINT

Patient	Lying supine with her body in side bending, her head and feet away from the operator and arms clasped across her chest.
Operator	Standing at the side of the plinth.
Principle	Assume the left ilium to be located in a position relatively anterior to the sacrum at the level of the sacro-iliac joint.
Technique	Cupping the patient's anterior superior iliac spine in the palm of his right hand, the operator reaches around the patient's shoulder girdle and rotates her thorax forward with his left arm, while restricting pelvic movement with his right hand.

SACRO-ILIAC JOINT

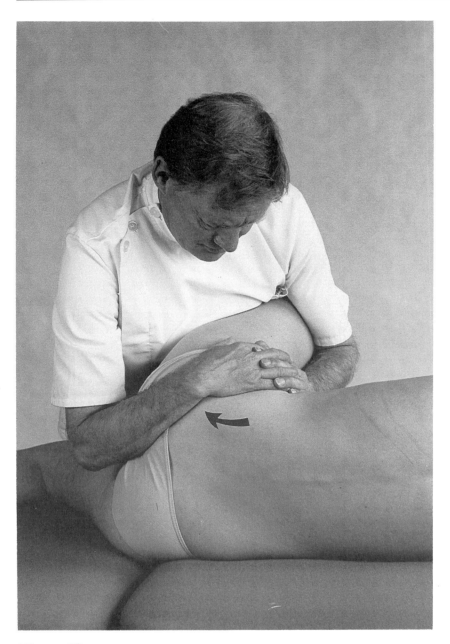

Plate 48
MOBILISATION OF THE SACRO-ILIAC JOINT

Patient	Side lying, facing the operator.
Operator	Standing at the side of the plinth, with the patient's upper thigh supported on his iliac crest.
Principle	To rotate the ilium backwards on the sacrum.
Technique	With his fingers interlocked, the operator encircles the patient's iliac crest, with the anterior superior iliac spine resting in the palm of his left hand. By rotating his whole body, he moves the ilium posteriorly.

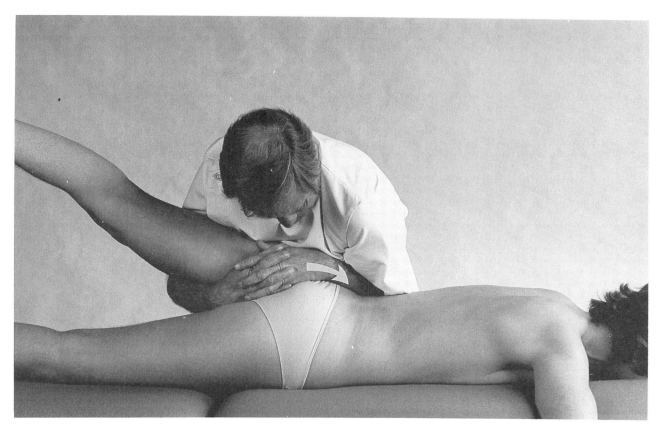

Plate 49
MOBILISATION OF THE SACRO-ILIAC JOINT

Patient	Lying prone.
Operator	Standing at the side of the plinth.
Principle	To rotate the ilium forwards on the sacrum.
Technique	With his fingers interlocked, the operator raises the patient's thigh into extension, adduction and internal rotation. He then exerts pressure onto the posterior iliac spine to produce a forward rotation of the ilium on the sacrum.

SACRO-ILIAC JOINT

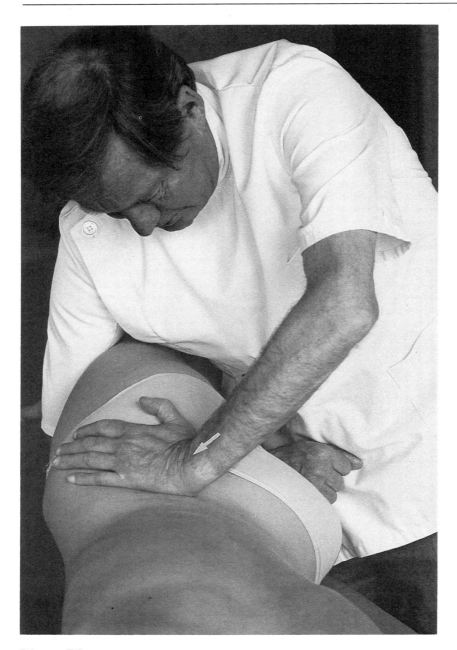

Plate 50
MOBILISATION OF THE SACRO-ILIAC JOINT

Patient   Lying prone.

Operator   Standing at the side of the plinth opposite to the sacro-iliac joint to be
               mobilised.

Principle   To rotate the ilium forwards on the sacrum.

Technique   With his right arm threaded between the patient's thighs so that a leverage
               is exerted upon the sacro-iliac joint, the operator presses the posterior
               superior iliac spine forwards and downwards.

SACRO-ILIAC JOINT

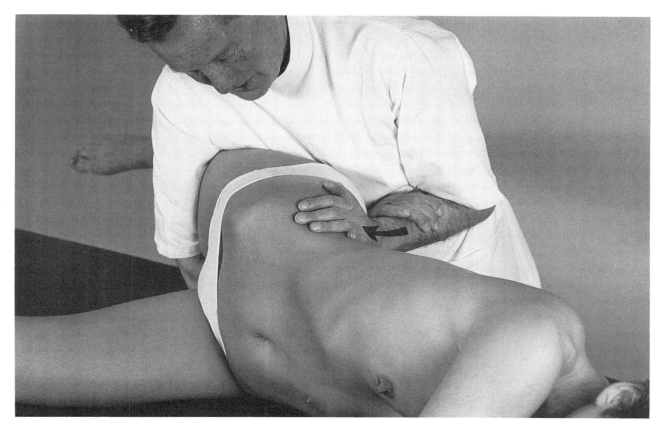

Plate 51
MOBILISATION OF THE SACRO-ILIAC JOINT

Patient	Side lying, with the lower hip and knee flexed in order to increase stability.
Operator	Standing behind the patient.
Principle	To rotate the ilium forwards on the sacrum.
Technique	The operator threads his right arm under the patient's upper thigh and grasps his left forearm. With his left hand pressed against the patient's posterior superior iliac spine, a rotational pressure is exerted around the arc of the iliac crest.

SACRO-ILIAC JOINT

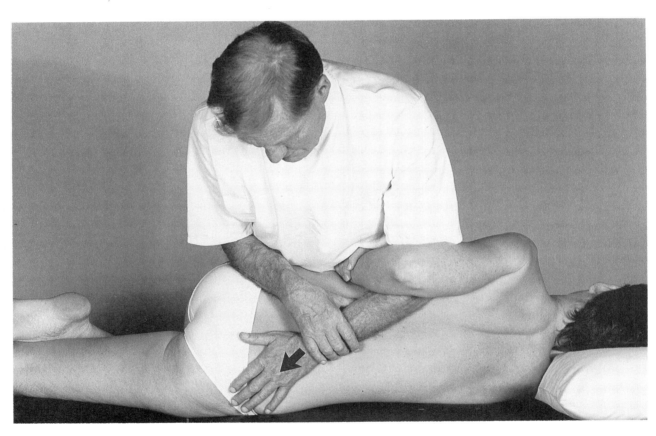

Plate 52
MOBILISATION OF THE SACRO-ILIAC JOINT

Patient	Side lying, facing the operator.
Operator	Standing at the side of the plinth.
Principle	To rotate the lower ilium forward on the sacrum.
Technique	The operator exerts a forward and downward pressure with the palm of his left hand onto the patient's right posterior superior iliac spine. Rotation of the pelvis is controlled by the operator's right forearm and abdomen.

THE
SHOULDER

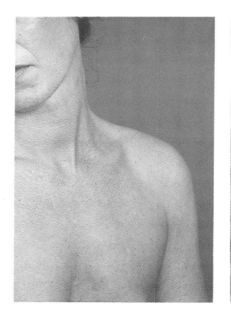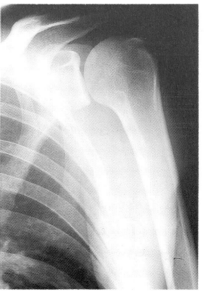

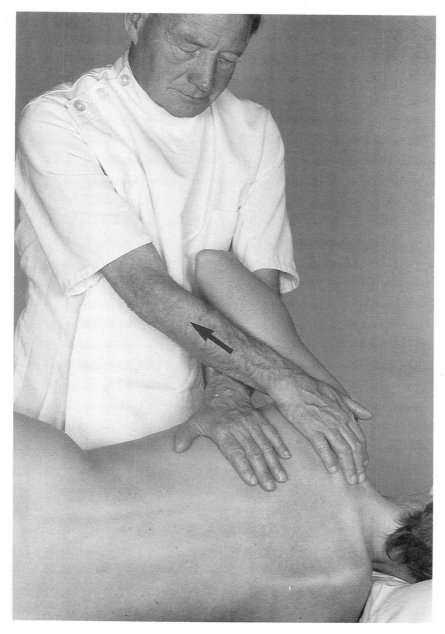

Plate 53
PASSIVE STRETCHING OF THE UPPER INTERSCAPULAR AREA

Patient	Side lying, with both knees bent.
Operator	Standing facing the patient.
Technique	With a cross-handed grip, the operator stretches the upper interscapular muscles. By a slight alteration of his grip and stance, he can apply the same technique to the middle and lower interscapular area, as depicted in Plate 54.

THE SHOULDER

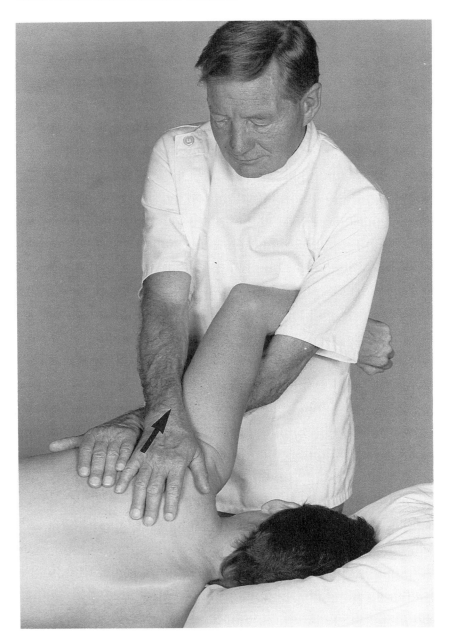

Plate 54
PASSIVE STRETCHING OF THE MIDDLE AND LOWER INTERSCAPULAR AREA

THE SHOULDER

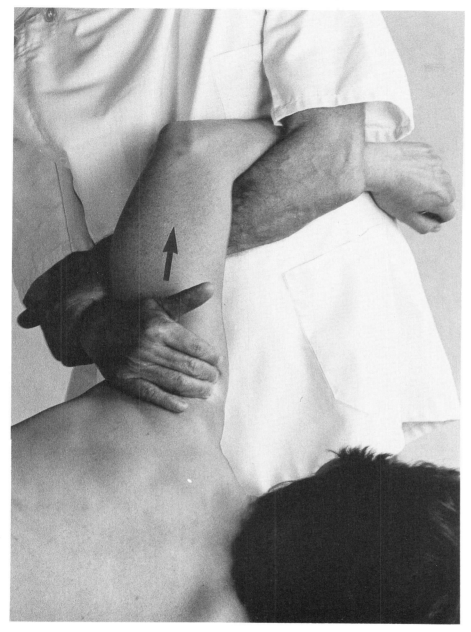

Plate 55
MOBILISATION OF THE GLENOHUMERAL JOINT

Patient   Side lying, with both knees bent, facing the operator.

Operator   Standing at the side of the plinth.

Technique The patient's arm is supported by a grip formed by the operator's left arm, the hand of which grasps his right wrist. By moving his body, traction, abduction and rotation can be applied to the glenohumeral joint. Note that the fingers of the right hand are free to palpate and localise the movement.

THE SHOULDER

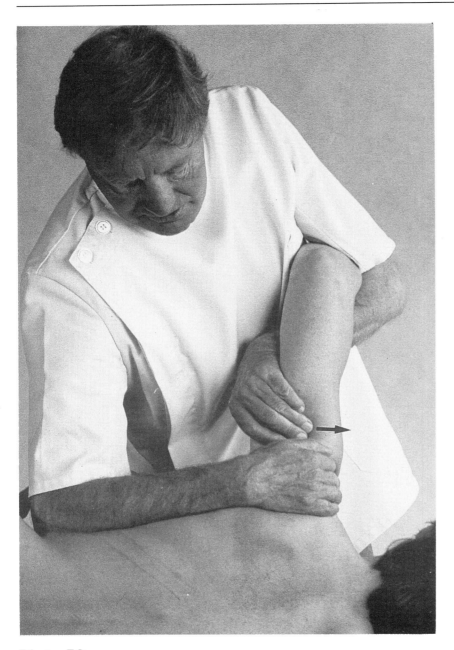

Plate 56
STRETCHING THE AXILLARY STRUCTURES OF THE SHOULDER

Patient   Side lying, with both knees bent, facing the operator.

Operator   Standing at the side of the plinth.

Technique With his right arm, hand and fingers, the operator fixes the angle of the patient's scapula and acromion process. The left arm then abducts the shoulder joint, at the same time allowing the fingers to palpate the axillary structures.

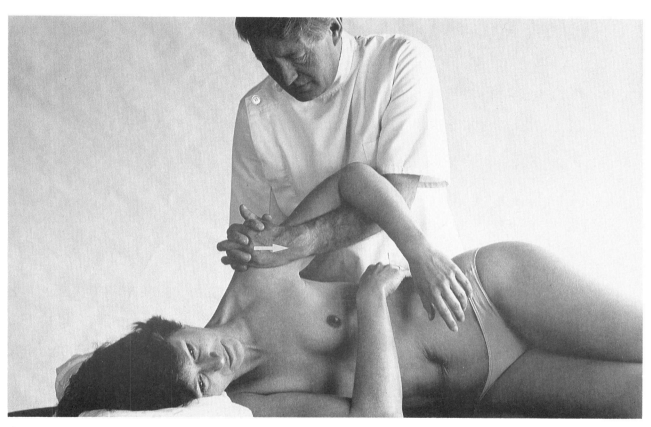

Plate 57
CAUDAL GLIDING OF THE HUMERAL HEAD

Patient	Side lying, with both knees bent.
Operator	Standing behind the patient.
Technique	With his hands clasped around the patient's shoulder, the operator slides his fingers off the acromion process onto the tubercle of the humerus and applies caudal traction.

THE SHOULDER

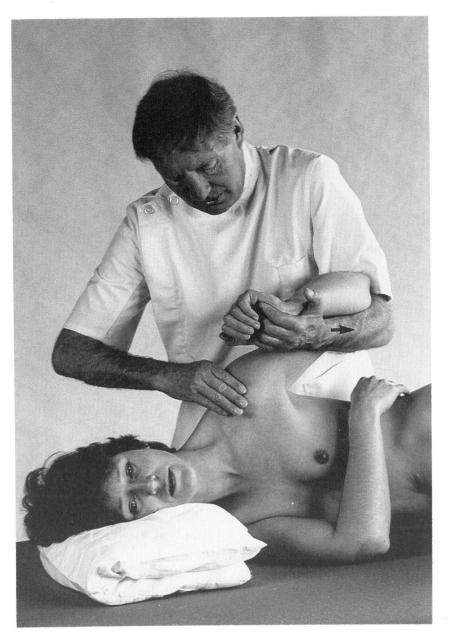

Plate 58
CAUDAL GLIDING OF THE HUMERAL HEAD

Patient	Lying with both knees bent.
Operator	Standing behind the patient.
Technique	The fingers of the operator's left hand are flexed into the patient's palm. In this position, various movements in the glenohumeral joint can be performed under traction. With his right hand, the operator palpates the joint.

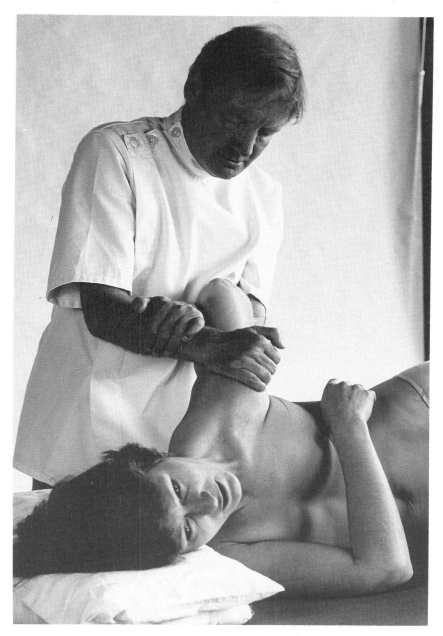

Plate 59
INTERNAL ROTATION OF THE HUMERAL HEAD

Patient　　Lying with both knees bent.

Operator　　Standing behind the patient.

Technique　　By grasping his own forearm, as depicted, the operator forms a comfortable cradle for the patient's arm, while allowing the fingers of his right hand freedom to palpate. Internal rotation of the humeral head may now be performed under traction.

THE SHOULDER

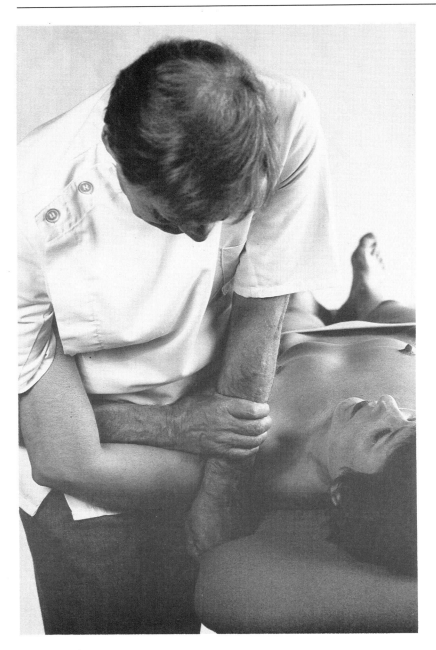

Plate 60
CAUDAL GLIDING IN THE GLENOHUMERAL JOINT WITH LEVERAGE

Patient   Lying supine, with her left arm over the side of the plinth.

Operator   Standing on the left side of the plinth.

Technique   The operator's left hand is fixed upon the plinth so that his wrist is in contact with the patient's shoulder. The patient's left arm is supported by the operator's right arm and thigh. By radial flexion of his left wrist, the operator exerts pressure on the tubercle of the humerus.

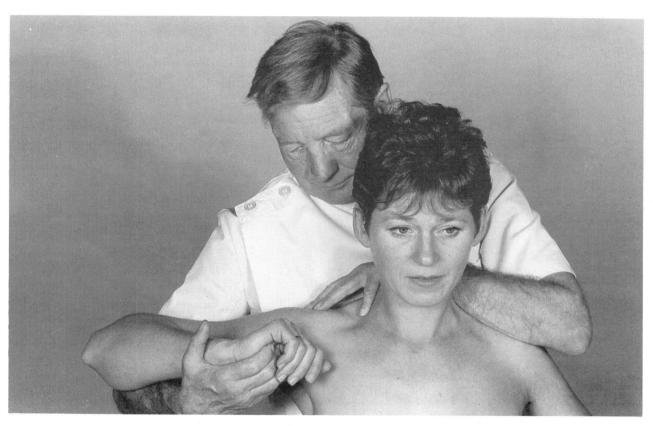

Plate 61
ROTATION IN THE GLENOHUMERAL JOINT WITH TRACTION

Patient   Sitting, with right shoulder in abduction and elbow flexed.

Operator   Standing behind the patient.

Technique   Supporting the patient's arm with his right forearm, the operator flexes his fingers into the patient's right palm. With this grip he can achieve all movements under traction, while his left hand is free to palpate the joint.

THE SHOULDER

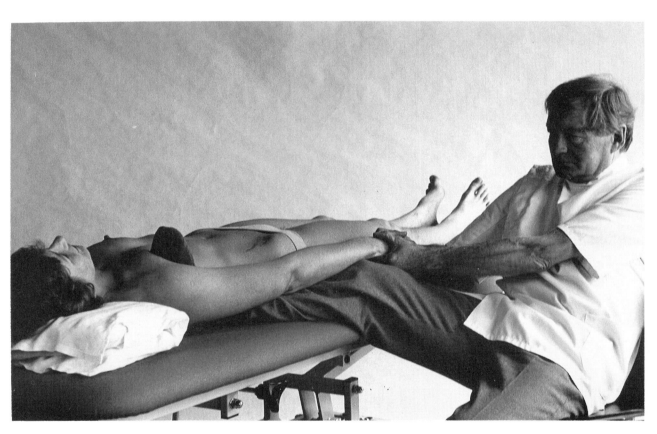

Plate 62
DISTRACTION IN THE GLENOHUMERAL JOINT

Patient	Lying supine.
Operator	Sitting at the side of the plinth.
Technique	The operator places his foot in the patient's axilla and grasps her forearm with both hands. By applying gentle traction to the arm and carefully adjusting the angle of his foot, the glenohumeral joint can be distracted.

THE
ELBOW

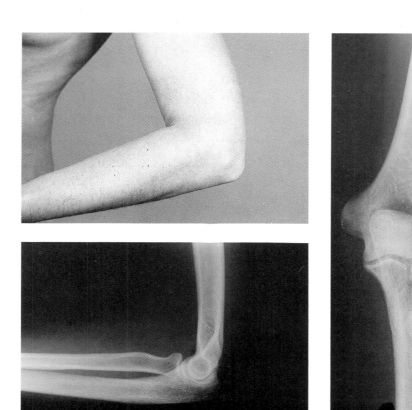

THE ELBOW

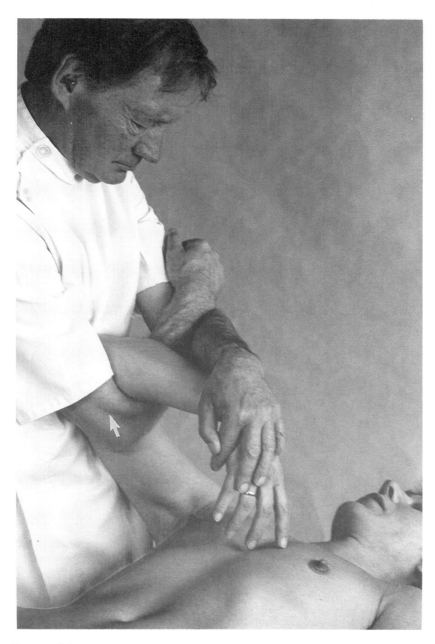

Plate 63
TRACTION TO THE ELBOW

Patient	Lying supine.
Operator	Standing at the side of the plinth.
Technique	To obtain an angle of flexion in the humero-ulnar joint in which separation of the joint surfaces is not restricted by either the olecranon or the coranoid process, the operator forms a tractional hold with the anterior surface of his own forearm against the patient's antecubital fossa. Minor adjustments can then be made by the operator's left hand.

THE ELBOW

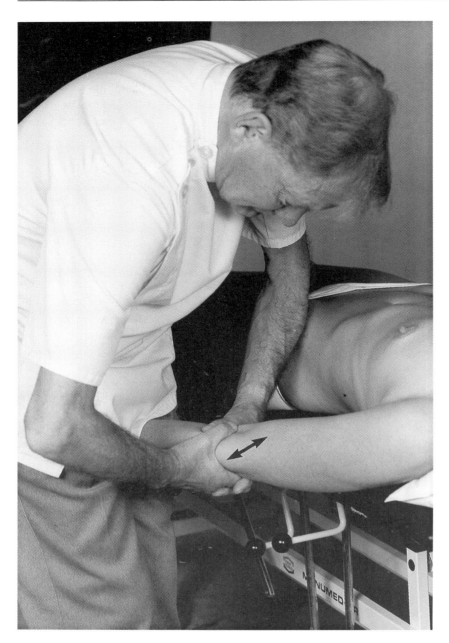

Plate 64
MEDIAL AND LATERAL MOBILISATION OF THE ELBOW

Patient   Lying supine.

Operator   Standing at the side of the plinth.

Technique   By supporting the patient's forearm between his knees and adding a few
               degrees of flexion to the elbow, the operator can obtain lateral and medial
               movement at the level of the joint.

THE
WRIST

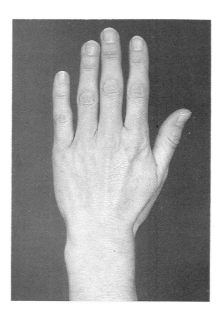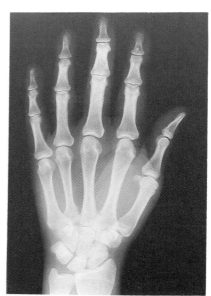

THE WRIST

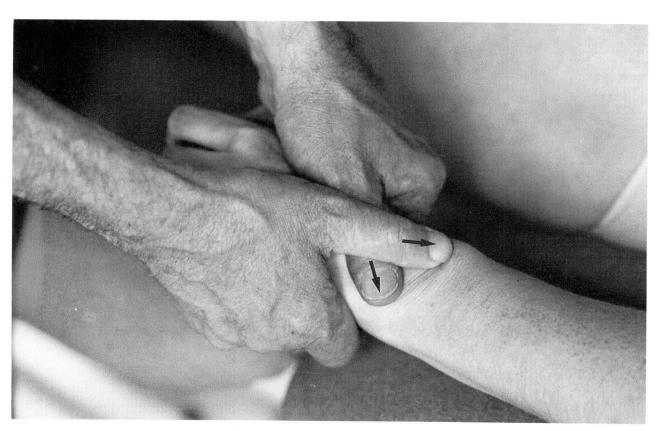

Plate 65
SPECIFIC MOBILISATION OF THE CARPAL JOINTS

Patient	Lying supine.
Operator	Standing beside the plinth.
Technique	By simultaneously adducting his thumbs and flexing his index fingers, the operator produces a separational effect which can be directed to individual intercarpal joints.

THE WRIST

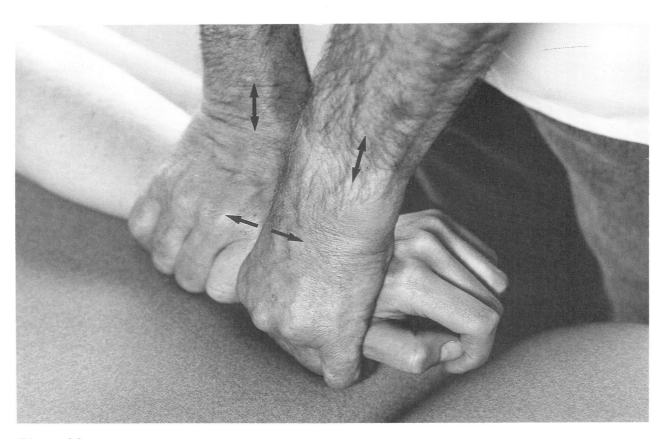

Plate 66
MOBILISATION OF THE CARPAL JOINTS

Patient   Lying supine, with her hand resting on the plinth.

Technique   By assuming the hold depicted, with his hands held in close apposition, the operator squeezes the patient's wrist, producing traction between the carpal bones. By moving his hands alternately in the vertical plane, specific dorsal and volar gliding movements can be achieved.

THE
HIP

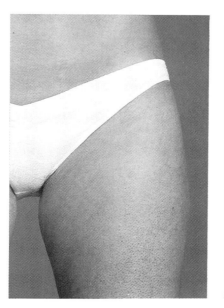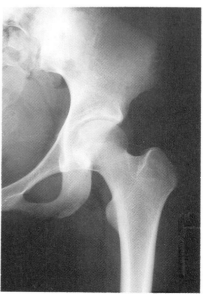

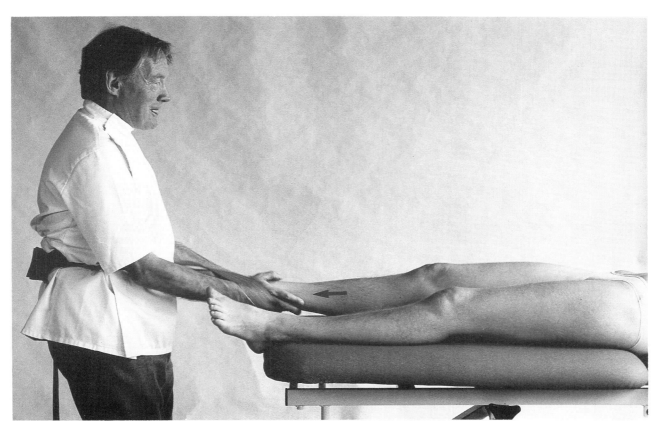

Plate 67
TRACTION OF THE HIP USING A STRAP

Patient   Lying supine.

Operator   Standing at the foot of the plinth.

Technique   With the strap describing a figure '8' around the operator's waist and above the patient's ankle, traction is applied by the operator leaning backwards. The strap should not come into contact with the patient but should be around the operator's hands.

THE HIP

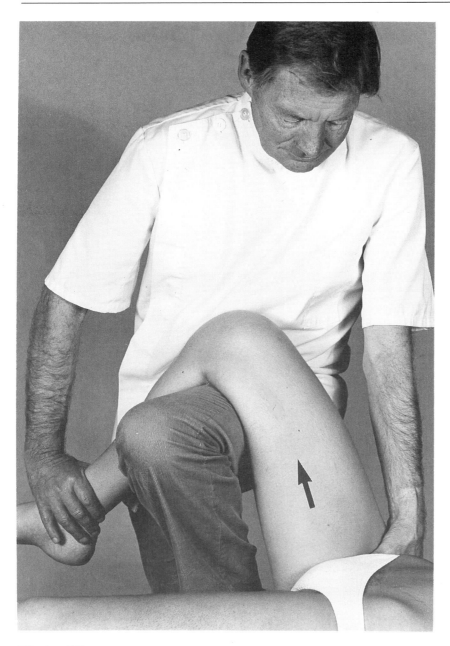

Plate 68
TRACTION OF THE HIP WITH ROTATION

Patient   Lying supine.

Operator   Standing with one foot on the plinth.

Technique   With the patient's knee bent over his thigh, the operator plantarflexes his ankle, thus producing traction in the hip. While the fingers of his left hand palpate the femoral triangle, his right hand rotates the patient's thigh.

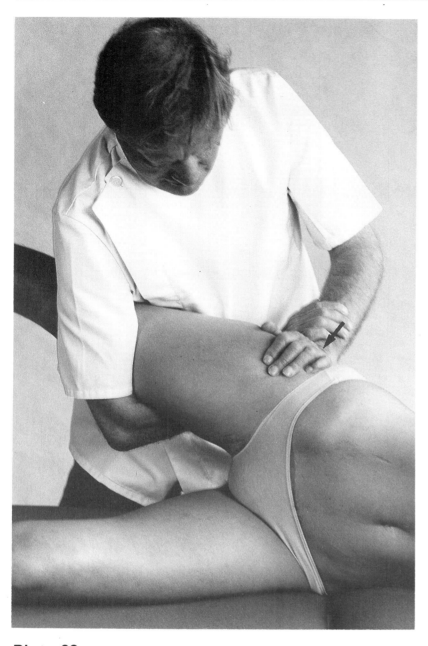

Plate 69
EXTENSION OF THE HIP

Patient   Side lying, with the lower knee bent.

Operator   Standing behind the patient.

Technique   By grasping his left wrist with his right hand, the operator forms a cradle
               for the patient's thigh. By transferring his weight, he brings the hip into
               extension.

THE HIP

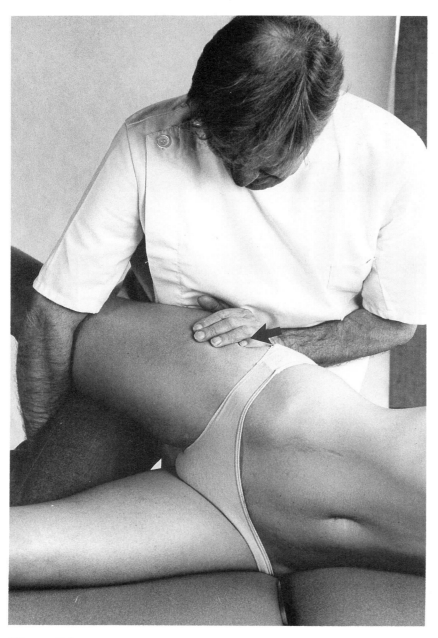

Plate 70
EXTENSION OF THE HIP USING LEVERAGE

Patient   Side lying, with the lower knee bent.

Operator   Standing behind the patient, with his right knee resting on the plinth.

Technique   By locking his right hand into the angle of his flexed knee, the operator effects a leverage against the patient's thigh. With his left hand, he presses forward onto the posterior aspect of the hip joint.

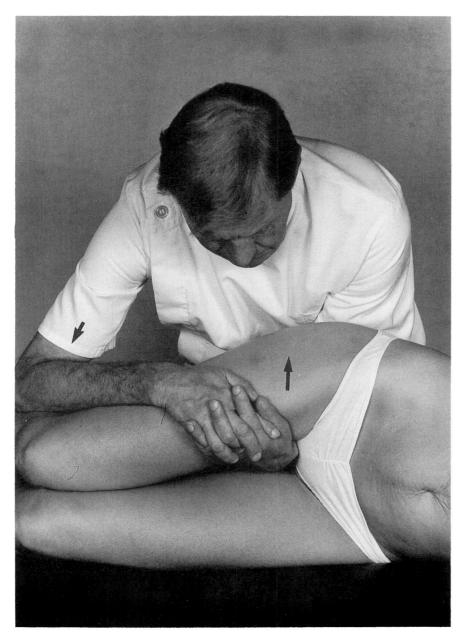

Plate 71
DISTRACTION OF THE HIP

Patient	Side lying.
Operator	Standing behind the patient.
Technique	Interlocking his fingers so that the anterior aspect of his forearm is in contact with the patient's thigh, the operator lifts with his clasped hands while simultaneously depressing the patient's knee with his elbow.

THE HIP

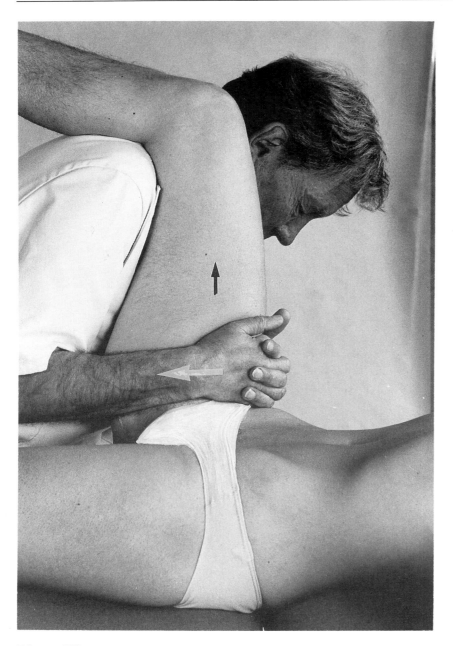

Plate 72
MOBILISATION OF THE HIP IN FLEXION BY TRACTION

Patient   Lying supine.

Operator   Standing at the side of the plinth.

Technique With the patient's flexed knee over his shoulder and interlocking his
fingers around the thigh, the operator produces a combination of vertical
and horizontal traction to which rotation can be added.

THE KNEE

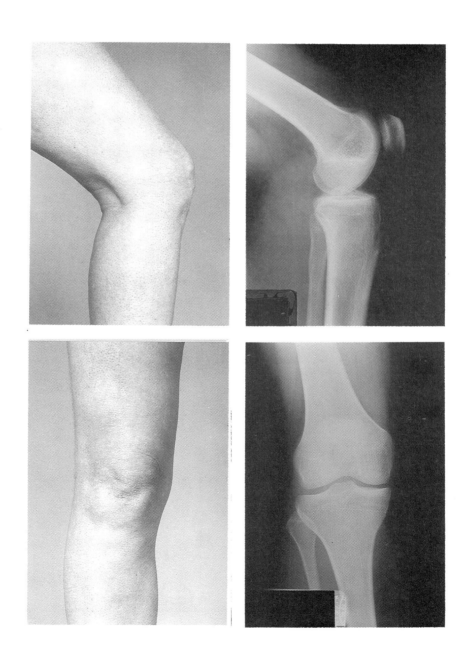

THE KNEE

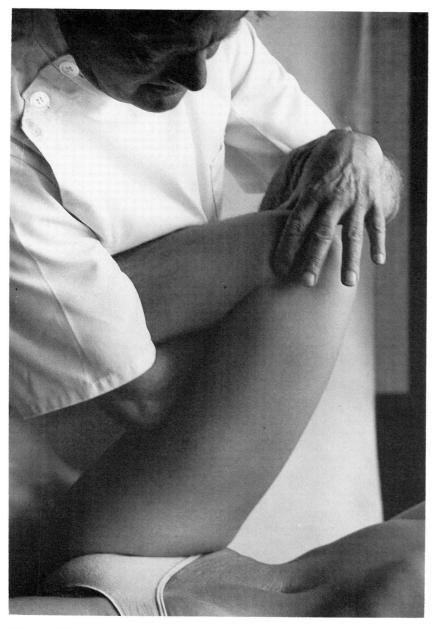

Plate 73
FLEXION OF THE KNEE USING A TWO-HANDED GRIP

Patient   Lying supine.

Operator   Standing at the side of the plinth.

Technique By threading his right arm through the patient's flexed knee and grasping his left forearm, the operator produces a comfortable cradle to take the weight of the patient's leg. The right hand is now free to palpate the joint.

THE KNEE

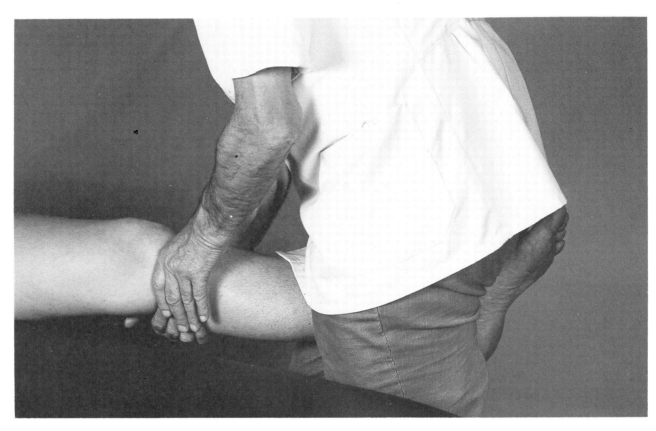

Plate 74
SIDE GLIDING OF THE KNEE

Patient   Lying supine.

Operator   Standing at the side of the plinth with the patient's lower leg supported between his thighs.

Technique   Grasping the knee around the joint line and adding a litte flexion, the operator induces a medial and lateral gliding in the joint.

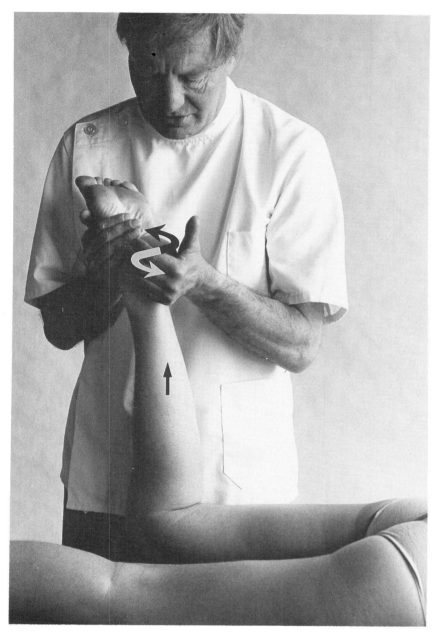

Plate 75
ROTATION OF THE KNEE

Patient	Prone lying.
Operator	Standing at the side of the plinth.
Technique	Grasping the patient's ankle with both hands and raising the knee clear of the plinth, the operator rotates the foot in both directions in various degrees of flexion.

THE KNEE

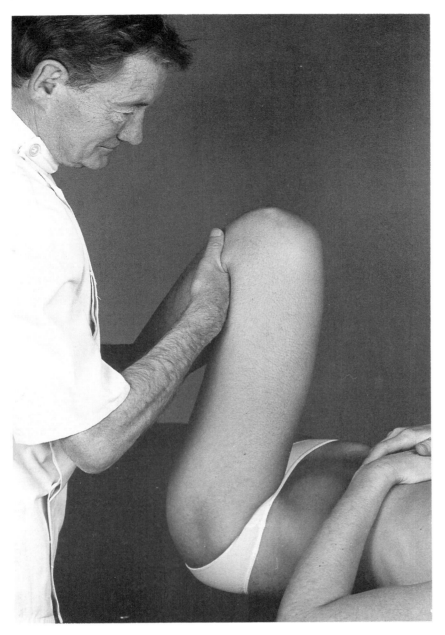

Plate 76
MOBILISATION OF THE SUPERIOR TIBIOFIBULAR JOINT

Patient   Lying supine.

Operator   Standing at the side of the plinth.

Technique   The operator gently flexes and externally rotates the knee onto his first metacarpophalangeal joint which acts as a fulcrum against the head of the fibula. The result is an anterior movement of the head of the fibula on the tibia.

THE
ANKLE

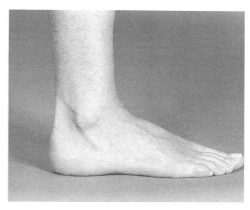

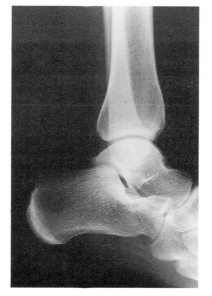

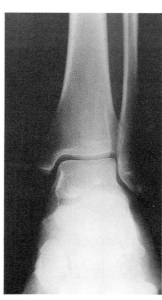

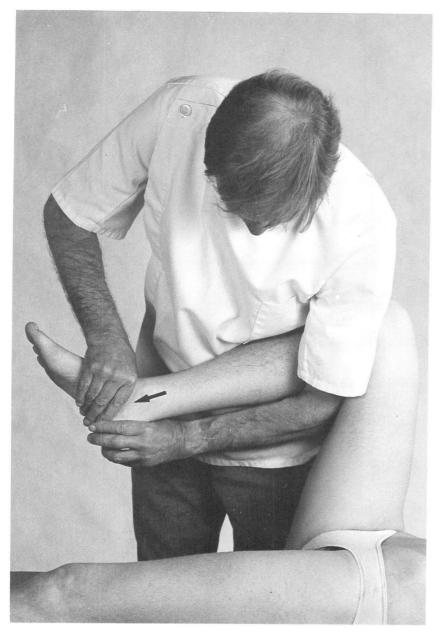

Plate 77
MOBILISATION OF THE ANKLE WITH TRACTION

Patient   Lying supine.

Operator   Standing at the side of the plinth.

Technique   The operator's left hand grips the patient's calcaneum and his elbow rests in the flexure of her knee. His right hand grasps the anterior aspect of the ankle. By transferring his weight towards the head of the plinth, traction is obtained in the joint; mobilisation in all directions is now possible.

THE ANKLE

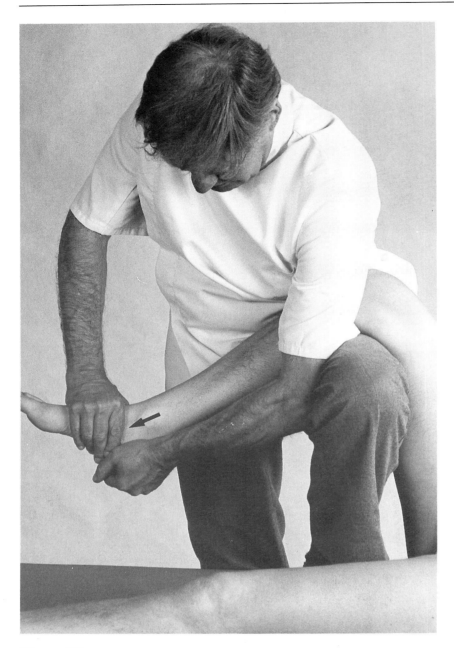

Plate 78
MOBILISATION OF THE SUBTALAR JOINT WITH TRACTION

Patient   Lying supine.

Operator   Standing with one foot on the plinth.

Technique The operator's left hand grasps the calcaneum while his elbow rests against his own thigh. The right hand maintains the foot in dorsiflexion and fixes the head of the talus. Traction is obtained by the operator transferring his weight towards the patient's head.

THE
FOOT

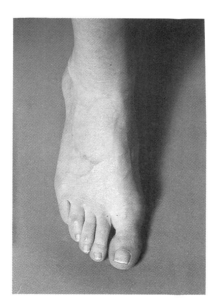

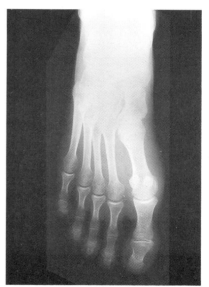

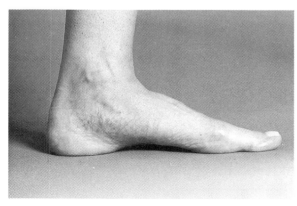

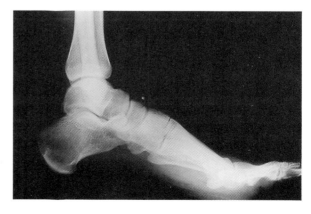

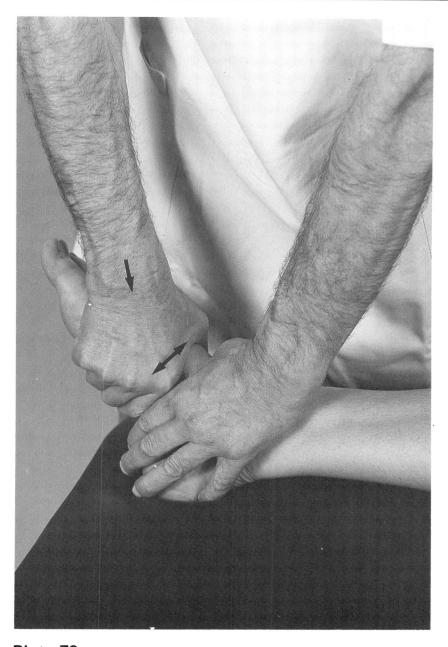

Plate 79
MOBILISATION OF THE TALONAVICULAR JOINT

Patient	Lying supine.
Operator	Standing at the side of the plinth.
Technique	Stabilising the talus with the left hand, the operator applies vertical compression along the shaft of the first metatarsal, cuneiform and navicular bones with his right hand. Gliding movements can be effected in the talonavicular joint.

THE FOOT

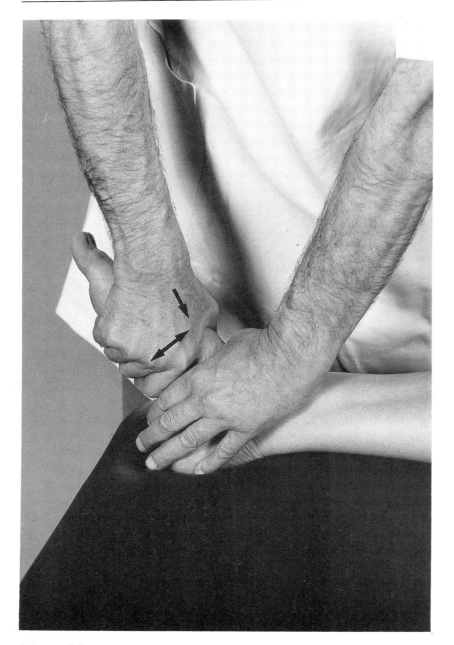

Plate 80
MOBILISATION OF THE CUNEONAVICULAR JOINT

Patient	Lying supine.
Operator	Standing at the side of the plinth.
Technique	Stabilising the navicular bone with the left hand, the operator applies vertical compression along the shaft of the first metatarsal bone with his right hand and grasps the cuneiform bone between his thumb and first finger. Gliding movements can be effected in the cuneonavicular joint.

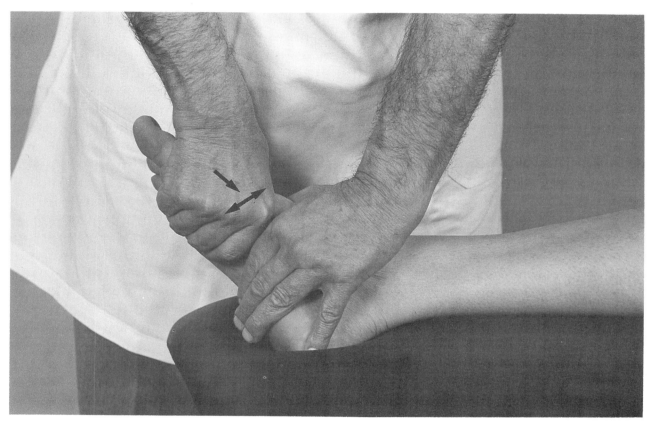

Plate 81
MOBILISATION OF THE TARSOMETATARSAL JOINT

Patient	Lying supine.
Operator	Standing at the side of the plinth.
Technique	Stabilising the cuneiform bone with his left hand, the operator applies vertical pressure along the shaft of the first metatarsal bone with his right hand. He then produces gliding movements in the tarsometatarsal joint.

THE FOOT

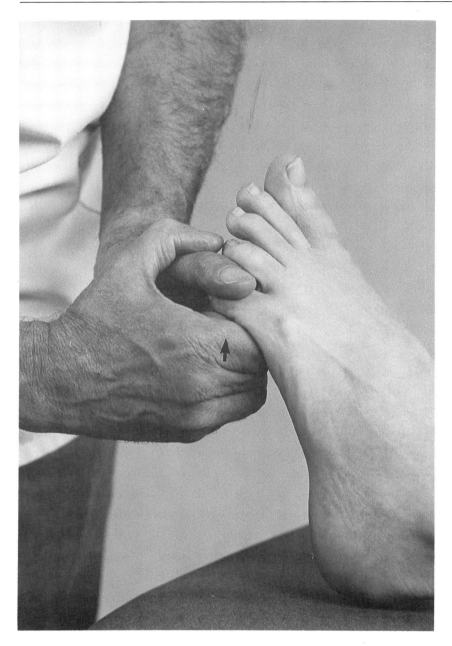

Plate 82
MOBILISATION OF METATARSOPHALANGEAL JOINTS

Patient   Lying supine.

Operator   Standing at the foot of the plinth.

Technique Gripping the toe between the thumb and first finger of one hand and
             reinforcing the grip with the other hand, the operator lifts both hands thus
             producing traction to the metatarsophalangeal joint.

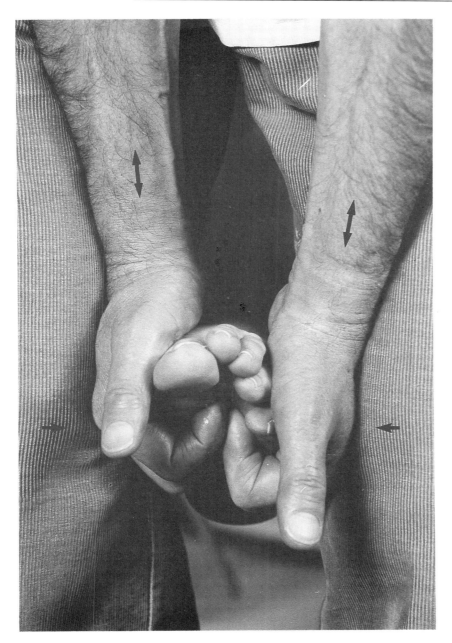

THE FOOT

Plate 83
MOBILISATION OF THE METATARSAL ARCH BY COMPRESSION

Patient	Lying supine with the leg over the edge of the plinth.
Operator	Standing beside the plinth, with his back to the patient.
Technique	Grasping the foot, as depicted, the operator compresses his hands between his knees. He then generates vertical movement from his shoulder girdle by alternately raising and lowering his hands, mobilising each element of the arch separately.

THE FOOT

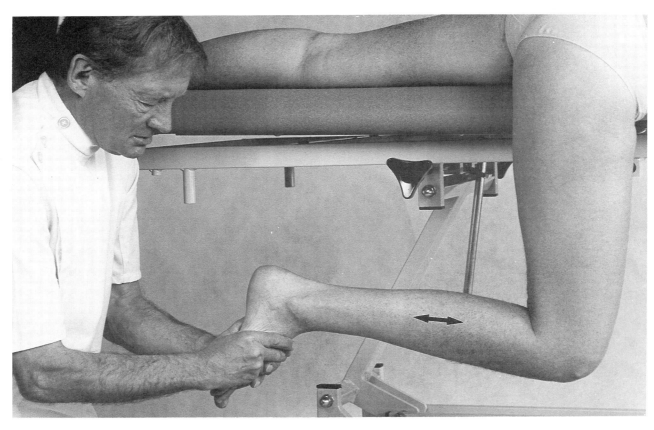

Plate 84
MOBILISATION OF THE CUBOID BONE

Patient   Prone lying, with the leg suspended over the side of the plinth.

Technique   Placing both thumbs on the inferior aspect of the cuboid bone, the operator sets up an oscillatory motion in the patient's leg, with the tibia travelling forwards and backwards parallel to the ground. At some point the momentum is suddenly aborted by the crossed thumbs, producing a whiplike effect against the cuboid bone. The ankle should be maintained in dorsiflexion.